Pregnancy and Pa

The views and experiences
in public care

Judith C   yo

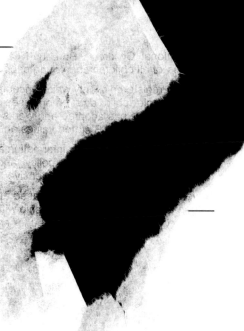

004

Published by National Children's Bureau Enterprises, the trading company for the National
Children's Bureau, 8 Wakley Street, London EC1V 7QE, Registered Charity number 258825.

ISBN 1 900990 42 3

© National Children's Bureau, 1999

Typeset by LaserScript Ltd, Mitcham, Surrey CR4 4NA

Printed by Biddles, Guildford GU1 1DA

Contents

List of tables		iv
Acknowledgements		vi
1	Introduction	1
2	Relationships with adults	21
3	Relationships with peers	44
4	Information about relationships, sex and contraception	57
5	Future aspirations	85
6	Pregnancy and decision making	103
7	Parenthood: expectations and preparation	125
8	Support for young parents	149
9	Support: accommodation and education	163
10	Summary and conclusions	183
References		194
Appendix A: Research design, methods and sampling		200
Appendix B: Additional tables		213
Index		217

List of tables

1.1 Age of component 2 respondents   18

1.2 Ethnic origin of component 2 respondents   19

1.3 Faith group of component 2 respondents   19

2.1 When you think of family life do you think of ...   22

2.2 Relationships with parents   24

2.3 Description of parents' behaviour   33

2.4 Description of carers' behaviour   34

2.5 People understanding, trusting, listening to and respecting
     the ideas of young people   40

3.1 Percentage of respondents who have a special friend
     they can talk to about personal things   45

3.2 Age at which it's all right for girls to start having sex   48

3.3 Age at which it's all right for boys to start having sex   49

3.4 Thinking about people under 16 do you agree that sexual
     intercourse is ...   49

3.5 Pressure on girls to have a boyfriend   50

3.6 Pressure on boys to have a girlfriend   51

5.1 In four years' time would like to ...   90

5.2 Factors that young people thought might stop them getting
     a job they would like in the future   96

6.1 Do you think that teenage pregnancies happen for any of the
     following reasons?   105

7.1 Will you look after your children in the same way as your
     parents looked after you?   126

7.2   When you think about being a parent what does this mean to you?   127

A.1   Percentage agreeing with the following statements   213

A.2   Nikki and Kris vignettes   214

Acknowledgements

Many people have helped to make to make this report possible. First and foremost, our thanks go to all the young people who generously shared with us their thoughts, ideas, feelings and experiences knowing that others, and not they, might benefit in the future. We hope we have done them justice in what we have written.

The study was funded by the Department of Health and we are grateful to Dr Carolyn Davies for her help and support. We would like to thank all the members of our advisory group: those from the Department of Health who focused our minds, Nina Biehal and Rachel Thomson whose knowledge and experience benefited us greatly and Paul Dolan whose constant support both within the group and in the field made a substantial difference to our task.

At the National Children's Bureau, we are indebted to the Research Director, Ruth Sinclair for her support throughout and to Gill Frances Lenderyou of the Sex Education Forum for filling in the many gaps in our knowledge.

Kay Rufai and Sabina Collier worked hard transcribing the taped interviews and helping with the preparation of the final report. Thanks also are due to Rossana Perez del Aguila, Maria-Louiza Constantinadou, and Teresa Keane, students on the MSc course in Social Research Methods at the University of Surrey who helped with the project during their placements at NCB.

When devising the questionnaire we were very grateful to other researchers who kindly allowed us to borrow or adapt their questions.

During the course of the fieldwork a number of local authorities, social services departments, leaving and after care services, children's residential homes, schools and individuals gave enthusiastic support. We are indebted to them for their interest and commitment.

1   Introduction

During the 1990s teenage pregnancy and parenthood have been afforded increasing prominence in Government policies and initiatives and, consequently, in media coverage. Subsequent debates appeared pulled towards the reiteration of negative stereotypes about young single mothers and pregnant schoolgirls while attempts to understand and explain their position were both scarce and under-reported. To those who looked beneath the surface it became clear during this time that certain individuals and groups were more prone to early pregnancy and parenthood than others and that among these were young women in or leaving public care. As a result this study was undertaken, with funding from the Department of Health, to explore the views and experiences of pregnancy and parenthood of young people in public care.

When the study began in 1995 it was within the context of four background factors. Firstly, there was a growing emphasis being directed by politicians and the media towards teenage mothers within the general debate about lone parents. Secondly, specific targets had been established within the *Health of the Nation* initiative to reduce the number of unwanted teenage pregnancies (Department of Health, 1992). Thirdly, findings from research indicated that high proportions of young women leaving care were pregnant or already mothers. Fourthly, the Children Act 1989, implemented in 1991, had made clear the duties of local authorities to advise and support young people whom they looked after on health and relationship issues, and to prepare them for adult life, one aspect of which might be parenthood.

After the project began a plethora of reports, policies and initiatives appeared on the two themes, teenage parenthood and the care system, which underpinned the study. A directive on the need for local authorities to listen to the views of young people themselves when planning services for them (Department of Health, 1996) appeared soon after we began seeking the views of young women in the care system. Two influential reports on the situation of children and young people looked after by local authorities (Utting, 1997; House of Commons, 1998) and a further one directed specifically at care leavers (Department of Health, 1997a) were followed by *Quality Protects* (Department of Health, 1998a), the Government's initiative to improve local authority services for children.

One of its stated aims is to ensure that the number of pregnancies to girls under 16 in public care does not differ from that in the general population.

During the course of the study the subject of teenage pregnancy remained firmly on the national agenda, even though the specific targets for reducing teenage conceptions within a national health policy framework (Department of Health, 1992) were dropped in favour of local target setting within the Green Paper *Our Healthier Nation* (Department of Health, 1998b). *New Ambitions for Our Country: A New Contract for Welfare* (Department of Social Security, 1998) set as one of its success measures a decrease in the rate of conceptions among girls under 16 in the areas with high rates. The subsequent Government Green Paper, *Supporting Families* (Home Office Ministerial Group on the Family, 1998), addressed ways of 'tackling teenage parenthood' and the *Independent Inquiry into Health Inequalities* (Acheson, 1998) highlighted the socioeconomic risk factors leading to disparities in the rates of unintended teenage pregnancy. In 1997 a National Task Group was established to explore unwanted and unintended teenage pregnancy (Health Education Authority, 1998). In 1998 their task was taken on by the Social Exclusion Unit, which had been directed by the Prime Minister to suggest strategies to reduce the rates of teenage parenthood and to minimise the risk of social exclusion for teenage parents.

In this context, the aim of this book is not only to offer insights into directions for future policy in relation to young people in public care in particular, but also to offer a contribution to the wider debate around adolescent parenting. The book is structured to indicate the potential for interventions at a number of levels, starting with the provision of sex and relationships education and moving through to the tertiary stage of intervention and support for young parents.

This opening chapter continues with a review of the relevant literature, and an outline of the study.

Young people looked after by local authorities

The Children Act 1989 provided for a range of court orders for situations where a child or young person needs protection from his or her parents or a secure substitute family. Such children and young people fall into three main groups:

- those accommodated under a voluntary agreement with their parents (Section 20);
- those who are the subject of a care order;
- those who are compulsorily accommodated such as those on remand.

'In care' now has a specific meaning and covers only those children subject to a care order. For more general use it was replaced by the term 'looked after' which covers all the above, although recently 'in public care' has come to be used interchangeably with 'looked after'.

The trend has been for fewer children to be placed in the public care system with numbers falling from 67,326 in 1986 to 51,200 in 1996 (Department of Health, 1997b). Official data on type of placement can only provide a snapshot on a particular day: some children will have experienced different types of placement at some stage of their care history; some children will move in and out of the care system; others will be in public care for only short periods of time. In general the trend over the last decade has been away from residential care and towards foster care and on 31 March 1996 the majority of children (65 per cent) were in foster placements. The relative balance between foster and other placements changes with age: in 1996 72 per cent of 5–9-year-olds were in foster care, while only 65 per cent of 10–15-year-olds and 51 per cent of 16- and 17-year-olds were in this type of placement.

The health and welfare of young people in the public care system has risen up the agenda in the last few years. The Children Act 1989 places duties on local authorities to include health issues in the planning and review process, and to arrange for statutory medicals. As the Children Act was implemented, the report on children in public care was released and health promotion was given an even higher profile (Department of Health, 1991a). The report commented on the variable quality of health care given to looked after children, noting that, despite routine medical examinations, little attention was paid to issues of prevention and health education.

The Children Act specifically comments on the need for sex education. The guidance and regulations on residential homes (paragraphs 1.92–1.96) require that in addition to health checks:

> staff of the home should actively promote the children's health with advice on health risks, for example, alcohol, substance misuse, sexual relationships and HIV/AIDS (Department of Health, 1991b).

Volume 3 on family placements states that: 'The experience of being cared for should include the sex education of the young person' (9.48) and that: 'Those responsible for the sexual education of young people will need to bear in mind the particular needs of different young people' (9.50) (Department of Health, 1991c). The issue can be particularly complex as social workers and carers may find themselves working with children who have been sexually abused, and indeed with abusers who are children. Such issues present challenges to standard models of sex education even to those trained in its delivery.

The Children Act 1989 also greatly enhances the duties of the local authority to prepare young people for leaving care. Section 24 of the Act places a duty on local authorities to 'advise, assist and befriend young people in order to promote their welfare when they cease to be looked after' and 'to advise and befriend' certain groups up to the age of 21. Volume 4 of the Guidance accompanying the Act provides comprehensive guidelines to enable staff to help prepare young people for living independently. This suggests, among other things, the importance of 'enabling young people to build and maintain relationships with others, (both general and sexual relationships)' (Department of Health, 1991b, Section 7.45). Research on young people who have left care points to the ability to form good relationships as a key factor in positive outcomes for them (Biehal and others, 1995). *Quality Protects*, the recent initiative to improve the standards of care provided by local authorities for young people also emphasises the importance of continuing care for young people who are no longer looked after and sets as an objective 'to maximise the number of young people leaving care after their sixteenth birthday who are still in touch with SSD, or a known and approved contact, on their 19th birthday' (Department of Health, 1998a).

In recent years the poor outcomes for young people who have experienced the care system have been well documented, and particular attention has been paid to the extent to which these cast a pall over their future lives. A major area of disadvantage lies in their education which is given insufficient priority both by those who teach them and those who care for them, with young people living in residential care being especially at risk of receiving inadequate support and encouragement (Cleaver, 1996; Berridge and Brodie, 1997). They are more likely than those in the wider population to experience changes of school, truancy and exclusion, and to leave the education system prematurely and with few, if any, qualifications (Department of Health, 1995a). Their absence from school also means that they do not receive information about career opportunities or wider social issues (Garnett, 1992).

Due regard is not always given to the health needs of children and young people in public care (Cleaver, 1996) and their emotional needs are particularly likely to remain unmet (Sinclair, Garnett and Berridge, 1995). They are more likely to engage in risk-taking behaviours which include smoking and the use of alcohol, drugs and solvents (Cleaver, 1996; Department of Health, 1997a) but in terms of health promotion they are less likely than other young people to be given information (McGuire and Corlyon, 1997). There is also an apparently high incidence of attempted suicide and self-harm among the looked after population (Buchanan and others, 1993).

In consequence, those who leave care are inclined to feel rejected and disaffected (Triseliotis, 1995) and are prone to unemployment, home-lessness, poverty and law breaking (Action on Aftercare Consortium, 1996).

Teenage pregnancy and parenthood

The age at which women have their first child has been increasing steadily and is now almost 27 years, thus throwing into even sharper relief than previously those who have a child when they are very young. The latest figures (for 1996) show that in England and Wales 94,377 young women under 20 became pregnant. This represents a rate of 63 in every 1000 young women in that age group. Just over a half of all these conceptions are to teenagers aged 18 or 19. The pregnancies of slightly more than a third of those aged under 20 were terminated by abortion, leading to 59,518 maternities. These maternities are not synonymous with births to teenagers since many 19-year-olds who conceive are aged 20 when they give birth. Thus in the following year (1997) there were 46,316 births to mothers under 20, two thirds of whom were aged 18 or 19 (Office for National Statistics, 1998).

Pregnancy, maternity and motherhood are very different experiences and carry different implications for teenagers who are 14 or 15 from those for teenagers who are 17 or 18. Of particular concern has been the relatively high rate of conceptions to girls under 16, which increased during the 1980s. Although this has fallen slightly from a high point of 10.1 per 1000 13–15-year-olds in 1990 to 9.4 per 1000 in 1996, the White Paper *Health of the Nation* had sought to reduce this rate to no more than 4.8 by the year 2000, that is a reduction of slightly more than 50 per cent from its 1989 level of 9.5 per 1000 (Department of Health, 1992).

In 1996 8829 girls under 16 became pregnant, of whom 72 per cent were aged 15 (Office for National Statistics, 1998b). This age group experienced a rate of abortion of 4.9 per thousand (52 per cent), thus reducing the number of maternities to 4279. Furthermore, many 15-year-olds have become 16 by the time they have the baby and in 1997 there were just 1600 births to mothers under 16, 82 per cent of whom were 15.

Notwithstanding the media and political focus on adolescent mothers, teenagers today are far less likely to have a baby than was the case 30 years ago. In 1996, the age-specific fertility rate for women under 20 was 29.8 births per 1000 women in that age group in England and Wales, compared with 42.5 per 1000 in 1964 (Office of Population Censuses and Surveys, 1992). Overall the number of births to young women under 20 has fallen by 42,000 in the last 30 years.

Despite this overall fall, international comparisons indicate that the teenage fertility rate (birth rates per 1000 women aged 15–19 years) for England and Wales, closely followed by the rates for Scotland and for Northern Ireland, are higher than any in any other economically developed country with the notable exception of the USA (Babb, 1994). The England and Wales rate of 33.3 (1990) compared adversely with the low rates of, for example, the Netherlands and Switzerland at 6.4 and 4.6 respectively. Moreover many European countries effected dramatic reductions in their rates during the 1980s when Britain was conspicuously unsuccessful in this respect.

Moreover within England and Wales there is considerable variation in the rate of conceptions to under-16s according to district health authority data. For example, in 1995 when the overall rate stood at 8 per 1000 this disguised a range which reached 16.1 in one area and fell as low as 3.8 in another. Moreover, the areas with high rates of conception typically have low rates of abortion among the under-16s. The highest rates of conception are associated with the deprived areas of inner cities and thus suggest a strong link with social and material deprivation. Nevertheless few commentators choose to see poverty not only as a consequence but also as a cause or contributing factor in teenage parenthood (Selman, 1998).

As recently as 30 years ago most births to teenagers were within marriage whereas now the majority (89 per cent) take place outside marriage and to a far greater extent than in any other age group. However, of the 41,089 babies born to unmarried mothers under the age of 20 in 1997, more than two thirds were registered in the name of both parents and more than half of those making a joint registration used the same address for both parents (Office for National Statistics, 1998a). This suggests that a majority of young mothers are in a cohabiting relationship, although such relationships are not only more fragile than marriages but are also especially vulnerable to breakdown when they involve young couples (McRae, 1993).

Little research has been undertaken on the partners of teenage mothers or, indeed, on young fathers in general. However, official statistics (Office for National Statistics, 1998a) indicate that in 1997 there were 10,513 births to fathers under 20, the majority of which were outside marriage but registered in the names of both parents. Many babies born to teenage mothers also have teenage fathers and thus it can be assumed that a reasonable proportion of the 13,209 births registered only in the mother's name will also involve young fathers.

Young fathers typically have poor levels of education (Burghes and others, 1997) and thus they tend to be in unskilled and low-paid employment and unable to make a financial contribution to their children. Those who do not live with their partner and child are less likely to be in employment than those who cohabit (Moore and Rosenthal, 1993). However, many young fathers do wish to play a part in their children's lives (Speak, Cameron and Gilroy, 1997) though they are frequently unaware of their rights and responsibilities (Burghes, Clark and Cronin, 1997).

Factors associated with adolescent pregnancy and parenthood

There is a body of research which points to a number of different factors involved in high rates of adolescent pregnancy and the way that these may vary for different groups of young people.

Sex education

A major study of 37 countries found that adolescent pregnancy rates are lower in countries where there is a greater availability of contraceptive services and of sex education (Jones and others, 1985). A more recent study by the World Health Organisation (Baldo, Aggleton and Slutkin, 1993) indicated that knowledge of sex and contraception does not encourage or increase sexual activity among the young but may, in fact, be instrumental in delaying sexual activity amongst young people and in promoting safe sex. Yet there are still major deficiencies in the sex education that most young people in this country receive (Thomson & Scott, 1992).

While many young people would like their parents to be the main source of education in this area, such education rarely takes place and information is more likely to be acquired through friends (Balding, 1994). Parents are keen for schools to assume responsibility (Allen, 1987). However, the provision of formal school sex education in England and Wales is uneven in both quality and quantity (Sex Education Forum, 1992; National Foundation for Educational Research (NFER, 1993). It has also been criticised as being overly scientific, inadequate and ill timed (Ford, 1991; Mori, 1991; Thomson and Scott, 1991; Johnson and others, 1994).

As already highlighted, a significant proportion of young people being looked after are likely to be missing educational provision (Audit Commission, 1994; Department of Health, 1995a) and, consequently, any school sex education. Volume 4 of the *Guidance and Regulations* accompanying the Children Act 1989 recognises this gap in provision and states that looked after children and young people should be given sex education since 'sexuality will be one of the most potent forces affecting any young person in the transition from childhood to adulthood' (Department of Health, 1991b, Section 7.48).

Informed or uninformed choice

It is difficult to know the extent to which adolescent parenting is a result of ignorance or choice. Recent research and commentary in this area questions the assumption that adolescent parenthood is inherently negative and highlights the limited economic and educational opportunities available to many of the young women who became pregnant at an early age (Dawson, 1997; Coleman and Dennison, 1998). Kiernan (1995) found in an analysis of data from the National Child Development Study that low educational attainment was the most powerful single factor associated with becoming a young parent. Teenage mothers were also more likely to come from families with low socioeconomic status where financial hardship was reported. In addition, there was also an association between young parenting and having a mother who herself had given birth as a teenager.

Once a pregnancy is discovered cultural, class and family factors may exert a powerful influence upon the decision to have and keep the baby

(Hudson and Ineichen, 1991; Phoenix, 1991). Although adolescent pregnancies may often be unplanned, they are not necessarily unwanted.

A response to childhood experience

There is a body of American research indicating that sexual abuse increases the likelihood of early pregnancy (Dryfoos, 1990; Boyer and Fine, 1992). Young people who have experienced rejection, disruption or abuse within the family situation are likely to be emotionally and psychologically vulnerable in ways that may increase the appeal of early parenthood. Where young people are unable to access alternative means by which to acquire adult identities, parenthood may appear to provide a means by which to become grown up, needed and loved (Musick, 1993). Kiernan's analysis showed an association between emotional difficulties during childhood and young parenthood (Kiernan, 1995).

In an analysis of data drawn from a longitudinal study in Scotland, Sweeting and West (1995) explored the relationship between family structure, conflict and health behaviours. The young women least likely to have been pregnant by the age of 18 were those living with both biological parents. Less time spent with the family at age 15 was associated with early pregnancy, although the amount of family conflict was not.

Pawlby, Mills and Quinton (1997) explored opposite sex relationship formation in girls aged 15–16 years. The research team matched a sample of 50 young women known to a social services department in an inner city location with a matched sample from a school. Those in the high-risk group who had experienced severe difficulties in family relationships were more likely to see their relationship with a current boyfriend as occupying a salient position in their network of friendship, spending more time with him than other friends, and having the expectation of a future cohabiting relationship. The researchers concluded that the identification of differences within and across groups is essential if we are to understand the path of early opposite-sex relationships.

The experience of public care

Certain groups of young people such as those who are homeless or who are in or leaving public care also appear to be more vulnerable to early pregnancy. Research on care leavers has pointed to high proportions of young women who are pregnant or have a child when they move on. In the study undertaken by Biehal and others (1992) nearly a quarter of the female sample were either pregnant or already a mother when they moved to independence or were legally discharged from care, while in Garnett's study of young women one in seven was in this position when they left care (Garnett, 1992). Moreover, in their further study Biehal and colleagues found that almost half of the women in their sample already had a child within 18–24 months of leaving care (Biehal and others, 1995). This contrasted markedly with the 5 per cent of all young women who at that point in time had had a child by the time they were 20. All these studies, however, had as their sample young people over 16 years of age. Little is known about younger people who are being looked after and who become pregnant or parents.

Preparation for adult life and parenthood

Parenthood is only one possible choice for young people as they move towards adulthood. Hence preparation for adulthood must be broadly based, especially if young people are more likely to choose parenthood when the range of options open to them is limited.

All schools are required by law to provide a curriculum that prepares pupils for the opportunities, responsibilities and experiences of adult life. But a recent review of parent education (Pugh, De'Ath and Smith, 1994) shows that the demands of the National Curriculum may have squeezed out this provision. However, the Department for Education and Employment White Paper *Excellence in Schools* (Department for Education and Employment, 1997) referred to parent education and the issue is currently being addressed by the Personal Social and Health Education (PSHE) Advisory Group, chaired by Ministers for Health and Education.

Even if parenting education were routinely provided, young people looked after by a local authority are the most likely to be disadvantaged: as we have already noted they are more likely to be out of school through truanting or exclusion than their peers who are not in public care.

Support for young parents

Current discourse has placed the issue of teenage parenthood within a framework defined by social problems, whether in relation to housing, lone parenting or the benefit system. The debate has also tended to focus on interventions at the primary level of prevention, that is how to reduce teenage pregnancy. However, the fact remains that almost half of under 16-year-olds and two thirds of 16–19-year-olds who conceive will continue with their pregnancy. It is therefore important to explore how agencies can intervene to reduce the health, social and economic consequences for mother and child.

Research studies show that in coping with birth and the transition to parenthood, key factors in the outcomes of pregnancy include how the experience is managed and the available network of friends, family and professionals (Pugh, De'Ath and Smith, 1994). A review of effectiveness of interventions in teenage pregnancy suggests that the following areas need to be explored (NHS Centre for Reviews and Dissemination, 1997):

- antenatal care;
- social support and parenting;
- pre-school education and support;
- parental education and support.

A review of antenatal support and education (Combes and Schonveld, 1992) noted that there are key groups who are less well served by professionals than others. They noted that young women tend to under use health services, booking late for antenatal care, and with poorer attendance at antenatal classes. Combes and Schonveld suggested that this is not a reflection of reckless disregard for the welfare of their child, but rather a reflection of embarrassment, ignorance of their pregnancy, lack of confidence, and lack of relevance of standard antenatal and parenting education to their circumstances.

Low service usage is of importance given that early motherhood is associated with poorer health outcomes for both mother and child:

- Babies born to mothers under the age of 20 are more likely to die in the first year of life (Office of Population Censuses and Surveys, 1997).
- Young mothers experience higher than average obstetric and postnatal complications, although this is likely to be associated with socio-economic factors rather the biological age (Makinson, 1985).
- While the nutritional needs of pregnant adolescents are unclear, there are concerns that this group is least likely to prepare for pregnancy due to poor diet (Garcia, France-Dawson and Macfarlane, 1994).
- Young mothers are least likely to breastfeed (Botting, Rosato and Wood, 1998).
- Smoking prevalence is likely to be high (Botting, Rosato and Wood, 1998) and, based on the available evidence, especially so for looked after young women (Parker and others, 1991; Polnay, 1994). Children born to women who smoke are believed to have an increased risk of sudden infant death syndrome, asthma, bronchitis and pneumonia (Garcia, France-Dawson and Macfarlane, 1994).
- There is a marked association between young age of the mother and low birth weight (Makinson, 1985). However, the babies of the youngest mothers, who are more likely to be living with family or friends, fare better in this respect than do those of older teenage mothers who are more likely to be living in the community without support (Botting, Rosato and Wood, 1998).

Osofsky, Hann and Peebles (1993) indicated that young mothers are more prone to depression than older mothers. Combes and Schonveld (1992) also noted that if young mothers are lone parents they are more likely to be experiencing lack of support and greater anxiety because of isolation or feelings of dependency.

In terms of parenting education, young mothers in particular may need support since the 'permitting circumstances' (Rutter, 1974) as they embark on parenthood are likely to be poor. That these mothers might need support in their parenting skills is not a reflection of their abilities, rather that the interaction of their economic, social and educational circumstances may make parenting more difficult.

Two pieces of research studies on young people leaving care to which we have already referred presented particularly disconcerting findings about the circumstances of young mothers and pregnant young women leaving care (Biehal and others, 1992, 1995; Garnett, 1992). These studies raised concerns about the support services that these young women received. A study of London boroughs indicated that only eight of 33 claimed to have any specific policies on young women in care who were pregnant or had children – and even then responses tended to be related more to practice than to policy – and only half had made any provision for them when leaving care (Bonnerjea, 1990). However, in all of these studies the issue of pregnant young women or young parents in care was incidental to much broader themes and therefore received limited attention.

Aims of the study

The available evidence pointed to the many background factors such as family status, educational attainment and childhood experiences that might predispose young people who are in or have been in public care to become pregnant or parents at an early age. Thus one aim of the study was to explore whether this subgroup of young people differed from their peers in the wider community with regard to their expectations of the future and their attitudes to sexual relationships and parenting. Equally important, however, was to promote discussion about the implications for services for the apparently high proportion of teenage mothers and mothers-to-be who were in or had recently left the public care system.

Three broad areas of focus for this study emerged: the preparedness of young people in public care for adulthood; an understanding of the choices that some of them make in becoming parents while still adolescent; and an examination of the support that young care leavers who are pregnant or parents receive from the care system.

Preparedness

If young people in public care are more likely to form opposite-sex relationships and have children at an earlier age than many in the general population then the level of their preparation for adult life would assume importance. We therefore sought to examine whether and how they had been prepared for adulthood and what education, formal or informal, they had received about relationships, parenthood, family life, sexual health and sexuality. A significant aspect of this was what young people themselves perceived to be their main sources of support and education in these areas. It was also important to establish whether any education they received took into account their specific life experiences, particularly when these included a history of parental rejection or abuse. Because young people in public care often experience frequent changes of placement we also wished to explore whether their formal education in the area of sex, personal relationships and preparation for adulthood had been affected by being looked after.

Recognising the importance to social workers and carers of operating within a policy framework, we also inquired whether local authorities had policies and practice guidelines in respect of sex, relationships and contraception for the young people they looked after.

Choice

A central theme of the study was young people's own experiences of parenting and family life and whether those experiences affected their own expectations, ambitions and choices. As part of this we were looking for any common reasons why young women in public care become pregnant and in particular whether such pregnancies result from choice or accident. In addition we wanted to find out how young women who have become pregnant unintentionally choose between abortion and continuing with the maternity.

Support

In terms of support our main focus was that given to young people being looked after who are pregnant or parents and any continuing support for those who have left the care system but are already, or soon become, pregnant or parents. While recognising that many local authorities address the needs of care leavers we wanted to establish whether they had written policies in relation to the preparation of young people for leaving care and for after-care services, and whether these included services for young people who are pregnant or parents. We were also interested in finding out whether these services and supports were adequate and appropriate in the young people's opinions.

A further important area was seen to be the role of social workers in helping young mothers and in particular whether there were any tensions between their role as supporter of a young mother in public care and that of surveillance over the care that she provided for her baby.

The study

Central to the design of the study was the wish to explore young people's lives through their eyes. Surprisingly few studies have explored young people's experiences of teenage pregnancy or of the public care system. The value of this approach was that it would offer an understanding of young people's lived experience of a setting and situation that few have experienced, as well as an insight into their views of relationships and of family life.

In addition, it was likely that the study would have clear policy and practice implications, and it is our belief that effective and efficient services can best be developed by involving the users of those services whether they be adult or child. In this case it was considered that an understanding developed from the young person's perspective might shed greater light on their needs and on appropriate intervention strategies both in preventing young women in public care from having unintended pregnancies and in supporting those who have children.

However, given the complexity of some of the issues involved it was considered that efforts should be made to collect contextual information from other sources. If useful feedback were to be offered to local authorities, information on policy and practice would have to be collected, and the role of social workers and carers understood. Nevertheless our focus throughout the study was the viewpoint of the young people themselves.

The research team were mindful of the ethical issues involved in conducting research with young people and especially that which involved sensitive topics (Alderson, 1995). Particular consideration was given to such issues as: consent from the young people as well as from adults; confidentiality and the action to be taken if information was revealed that a young person was at risk; the freedom for young people to opt into and out of the research; and the need to offer feedback to young people themselves.

The study was carried out in several local authorities in England between 1995 and 1998. It was divided into three discrete but interlinked components which sought to address the issues identified above. The two research components are described below and a third component, building on the findings from the research, was the production of a workbook for pregnant young women and young parents in public care (Mason and Lewis, 1999).

Component 1

The main focus of component 1 was the provision of services and support to young people who are pregnant or parents and who are being or have recently been looked after by a local authority. It was not intended to provide a representative picture of provision throughout the country but rather to locate the research in selected local authorities and to explore young people's experiences in the context of local policy and practice. Information was gathered using in-depth interviews as this method affords explanation and understanding of respondents' statements and takes into account the emotional issues involved. Contextual data were collected from professionals located in each social services department.

There were four main parts to this phase:

- Interviews with staff in 11 local authorities to gather information on local policy and practice in relation to looked after young people, sex education and support in parenthood and also to gain their cooperation in identifying and contacting young people.
- Thirty interviews with young people who were in or had recently left public care and who were or were about to be parents.
- Twenty interviews with social workers and carers linked to the young people above.
- Two case studies where a number of other key players, for example parents, were interviewed. An account of these is contained in the full report of component 1 (Corlyon and McGuire, 1997).

The initial selection of the local authorities was based on and dictated by many factors but one of our prime concerns was to obtain a geographical spread and a mix of local authority types and sizes. Of the 11 authorities involved in component 1 of the study, two were in the north-east, four in the north-west, two in the central area and three in the south. Seven authorities had a population size of under 250,000, three had between 300,000 and 1,000,000 inhabitants, and the remaining one over 1,000,000.

In each local authority social services department a link person was identified who was asked to provide information in the first round of interviews on the numbers of looked after young people within the authority who were pregnant or parents and on three broad policy areas as regards young people looked after: sexual behaviour and pregnancy; education about sex and relationships; and the transition out of care. Any plans for change by the authority were also discussed.

As it became apparent that most authorities did not maintain lists of young people who were pregnant or parents and who were still being looked after or were recent care leavers, the link person assisted in making contact with carers and social workers who were able to identify these young people. We were thus dependent on gatekeepers to access the sample.

Social workers or carers passed on to the young people who met the criteria for selection a letter from us explaining the research. Those who were agreeable to interview then had the option of either returning a form directly to the researcher or asking the social worker to establish contact on their behalf. The resulting interviews with young people were usually carried out in their accommodation, although three were conducted in after-care offices at the respondent's request.

Although it was important to cover the topics in the prepared interview schedule these were not dealt with in any rigid sequence nor were they exclusive. Other issues introduced by young people themselves were discussed. The aim was to make the exchange more akin to a conversation than a structured and formal interview. Interviews were usually tape recorded but notes were also taken since conversation was often in danger of being obliterated by noises from babies and children.

Once the interview with a young person was completed a social worker, carer or after-care worker most involved with that young person was identified. In some cases where the young woman was in her later teens there was no regular contact with a worker. These interviews were always carried out after those with the young person in order to avoid having any information and/or preconceived ideas before the young person's interview.

Component 2

The second component was located in two of the areas involved in component 1. Its focus was the way in which the differing experiences of young people might impact on future expectations, particularly in terms of relationships and parenting, and thus involved the comparison of young people in public care with those who lived with their families. This component consisted of two parts:

- questionnaires completed by 212 teenagers, half of whom were in public care;
- follow-up interviews with 67 of the questionnaire respondents.

Questionnaires were administered to two groups of teenagers, roughly equal proportions of boys and girls, the majority of whom were aged 14 and 15. Half the sample was in public, predominantly residential, care; in tables they are described as the 'looked after' sample and in the text the terms 'in public care' and 'looked after' have been used interchangeably. The other half of the teenagers in this component were living with their families and were mainly attending schools in the same areas in which the looked after young people lived. A very small proportion was drawn from a youth club. The group is referred to in the tables as the 'school' sample and in the text either by this name or as the 'comparator group'. The matched samples consisted of 106 questionnaires in each.

Quantitative methods offered the opportunity to explore whether the experiences of looked after young people in terms of the services they received and their attitudes to relationships and parenthood were significantly different from those of their peers who were not looked after.

In the three schools visited, the questionnaire was filled in during a Personal Social Education (PSE) lesson or form period, and in the youth club an early evening session was set aside. Although at least one teacher or youth worker was present on each occasion, a self-completion approach offered a degree of confidentiality. The researcher remained on hand to help with any difficulties that arose during completion of the questionnaire.

The situation for the looked after group was more problematic. The intention was that young people from residential care *and* foster care be involved and the lists supplied by the collaborating social services departments included young people in both types of accommodation. However, the logistics of contacting such a dispersed sample were daunting.

Time would not have permitted each young person to be contacted individually and a postal survey would have meant the researcher would not be on hand to assist where literacy was an issue, nor would this have achieved the desired response rate. Again a group-based approach to questionnaire completion was adopted. However, there was no natural point at which such young people spread across a large city might meet. Initial attempts to organise late afternoon or early evening events in conjunction with local health promotion and youth workers at various locations throughout the city met with only limited success. An out-cropping approach to sampling was subsequently adopted: the researcher made appointments at residential homes and those on the list who were at that address and who consented filled in the questionnaire. Although a more effective way of collecting data, it became more time consuming than anticipated with the researcher visiting 22 residential homes a maximum of four times.

Collection of the quantitative data was followed by personal and group interviews with 67 respondents, spread between the two samples. These interviews explored further some of the issues raised in the survey. The original intention had been to complete the collection of quantitative data and then select, from those who had completed a questionnaire, a number for the qualitative interview. However, given that young people in public care frequently change placement or leave the care system, there was no guarantee that young people involved in the quantitative stage would be contactable for an in-depth interview some time later. Therefore qualitative interviews with those in the looked after sample who had given their agreement were completed as soon as possible after the questionnaire had been filled in (typically one or two weeks later). They were not usually undertaken simultaneously with the collection of the quantitative data as this was considered to be too onerous for the young people. Exceptions were a few cases where a young person elected to fill in the questionnaire with the researcher and engaged in conversation while doing so.

In the school sample the respondents for the qualitative interviews were not matched with the looked after sample, but rather included all those young people who were willing to participate, who numbered 29 in total. Interviews took place on the school premises either at break times or within PSE lessons.

In both samples the qualitative data were collected by a mix of large and small group discussions and one-to-one interviews.

Tapes made during the in-depth interviews and group discussions in components 1 and 2 were fully transcribed and analysed. Data collected via the questionnaires were analysed using Statistical Package for the Social Sciences: descriptive and summary statistics were calculated and measures of association employed. Significance levels (P) were calculated using the chi-square test and a 5 per cent level of significance was used. In the tables illustrating the findings, the results from (a) all, (b) male and (c) female respondents in the two samples have been compared. Those results marked with an asterisk (*) indicate a significantly higher percentage than that in the comparable sample.

In discussing the findings, no names of local authorities or of individuals who participated are used in either the text or the quotes from interviews. This has been done to preserve the confidentiality that was guaranteed to all respondents.

Further details about the methods and data collection appear in Appendix A.

Sample details of young people

Component 1

Thirty-one young people gave agreement to interview and 30 were interviewed; one young woman had moved and no forwarding address could be obtained.

In terms of the individual interviews, respondents were not evenly distributed amongst the four regions that had been identified. The majority (14) were located in the central region, followed by 12 in the north-west, three in the south and one in the north-east. In addition to the interviews, three group discussions with young mothers were held. These were located one each in the north-east, central and south regions.

The respondents consisted of one young father and 29 young women who were either mothers or were pregnant. Of these, six were pregnant, 21 had one child and three had two children, including two who were also pregnant for the third time.

Seven were aged 16 or under, and 23 were over 16. Although the majority were over 16 at the time of interview most of the young women had been pregnant for the first time when they were aged 16 or under. These included young women who had had a previous abortion or a baby adopted. No interviews were conducted with young women whose sole experience of conception had ended in abortion or adoption. Social workers were asked only to identify young women who were either pregnant or mothers. Although theoretically young women who were pregnant but considering not keeping the baby may have come forward for interview, in practice this was extremely unlikely and none did so.

Although attempts had been made to select areas with a relatively high proportion of minority ethnic groups, there were very few respondents who were not white European. Young African Caribbean people, who are over-represented in the looked after population, did not have the equivalent representation in this sample. One person described herself as Asian, three described themselves as black and a further three said that they were of mixed parentage. The remaining 23 were white. The majority of their partners had the same racial origins as the respondents.

At the time of interview the young women had a variety of living arrangements according to their age and circumstances. Twenty were living alone either in some form of supported accommodation (nine) or in the community (11). Seven of the 'older' mothers were living with a partner. Only one young mother was in a foster placement.

The majority of young people were looked after on a voluntary basis: in total nine had, or previously had, a care or supervision order in effect. In terms of their care history, they fell into two distinct groups: those who had first been looked after in childhood and had not returned to their family of origin (just over one third of the sample) and those who had first been looked after in adolescence. Only four respondents came from families in which their parents were still living together.

Component 2

Although attempts had been made to involve young people living in foster care, most of the respondents in the looked after sample were in residential care at the time of data collection. The comparator sample was drawn predominantly from pupils in school year 10 in three schools and a small proportion was drawn from a youth club.

For both samples the mean age of respondents was 14.7 years and the modal age 15 years. Although the two samples displayed a similar age profile, there were slightly more 16-year-old respondents in the looked after sample than had been anticipated.

Table 1.1   Age of component 2 respondents

Age	Looked after % ($n = 106$)	School % ($n = 106$)
13	5	1
14	31	31
15	46	61
16	18	5
17	–	2

In terms of gender, the looked after sample was divided equally between males and females while the school sample comprised 56 per cent males and 44 per cent females.

No selection was made according to ethnic group but young people were asked to define their ethnic origin. While the two samples were reasonably well matched in terms of young people describing themselves as white, there was some imbalance between the minority ethnic groups represented, with a higher proportion describing themselves as of mixed parentage in the looked after sample, and a higher proportion from a Pakistani background in the school sample.

Table 1.2   Ethnic origin of component 2 respondents

	Looked after %	School %
White	70	69
Pakistani	–	12
Mixed parentage	18	5
Black Caribbean	8	8
Black African	2	–
Bangladeshi	–	1
Indian	–	1
Chinese	1	1
Other	2	3
Not known	–	–

It was considered that religious beliefs may possibly affect attitudes to the family and to parenting. For this reason, young people were asked whether they had been brought up to follow any religion. Eighteen per cent of the care sample claimed to be religious or very religious compared with 26 per cent of the school sample, although most (84 per cent of the care sample and 79 per cent of the school sample) claimed never to attend a religious or faith meeting.

Table 1.3   Faith group of component 2 respondents

	Looked after % (n = 96)	School % (n = 84)
Church of England	63	43
Catholic	14	23
Church of God	2	7
Pentecostal	1	7
Jewish	–	1
Muslim	–	13
Sikh	–	1
Other	3	2

Half of the care sample had been looked after for one year or less but the upper quartile was two years. The majority had entered the care system in their teens, with the modal age being 13 years. The number of placements experienced varied and, while 23 per cent had experienced only one placement, 33 per cent had experienced four placements or more and 11 per cent had had 11 or more. The longest time in any one placement also varied with an interquartile range of six months to two years. However, a small number of respondents had experienced a greater degree of stability and the length of the longest placement was 16 years.

Respondents were asked their opinions on the frequency of contact with their social worker. Eight per cent considered that they saw them too often, 41 per cent thought that contact was about right, and 51 per cent that they did not see them often enough. There was no difference in response by gender.

Further details about the samples in both components 1 and 2 appear in Appendix A.

2 Relationships with adults

A major aim of the study was to explore whether the experiences of young people in public care impact on their expectations of the future. An important factor in parenting styles and behaviour is the personal experience of being parented. The children of parents who themselves have been in the care of a local authority are more likely to be received into care than those whose parents have not (Bebbington and Miles, 1989). Whether this is the result of genetic disposition or learnt behaviour is unclear but we would anticipate that their own experiences, both good and bad, might impact upon their views of family life and how they intended to parent their own children. In addition those who have suffered family rejection or abuse might find more appeal in early parenthood than those who have not.

We begin by exploring the young people's experiences of and attitudes towards family life and then move on to look at the relationships they have with some of the significant adults in their lives. While we acknowledge that there may be other adults who are important to these young people (Marsh and Crow, 1998), for the purposes of this chapter 'significant adults' are confined to parents, social workers and carers. Where possible, we have tried to draw parallels with the relationships that young people in the wider community have with their parents.

Family life

The looked after sample as a whole had larger families than the school sample: whereas 40 per cent of them had more than two brothers and 33 per cent more than two sisters, the comparative proportions were 20 per cent and 16 per cent for the school sample.

Data from the qualitative part of component 2 indicates that the families of the looked after respondents were not only large but also complex with step-parents, step-siblings and half-siblings featuring strongly. Many reported having younger siblings, frequently from a parent's second marriage or relationship and, in common with the young women from component 1, thought that their care of these siblings, and nieces and nephews, would be a valuable experience to them as parents.

We considered it important to explore how young people who are being cared for away from home understand and make sense of family life. In component 2, young people were asked to select from a list of 12 options what they thought about when they contemplated family life. The results are set out in Table 2.1. If the answers are ranked in order of proportions agreeing with each definition of family life, there is little difference between the samples. Respondents from both were most likely to think of babies or young children and a couple with children and least likely to think of a lone father or step-parents.

However, there are some interesting points of comparison. While the proportions who included step-parents in their thinking were low, one quarter of the looked after sample did so compared with only one tenth of the school sample. The proportion including violence was twice as high in the looked after sample (29 per cent) as it was in the school sample and was indicated by more girls (35 per cent) than boys (24 per cent). Half the respondents in the looked after sample also included arguments in their thinking and again many more girls (56 per cent) than boys (46 per cent) did so. In respect of both violence and arguments the differences between the samples were significant. Children in the looked after sample were more likely than those in the school sample to associate watching TV with family life.

It is hard to know whether this is respondents' representation of their own family life or a picture of 'ideal' family life or a combination of the two. The high incidence of 'a couple with children' in the looked after sample is indicative of idealisation since that was clearly not their current situation:

Table 2.1   **When you think of family life do you think of ...**

	Looked after (%)			School (%)		
	Total	Male	Female	Total	Male	Female
Babies or young children	70	70	69	69.5	78	60
A lone mother	29	26	33*	21	24	18
A couple with children	79	82	77	82	86	78
A lone father	17	18	15	16	22	9
Step-parents	25.5*	26*	25*	10.5	14	7
Feeling content	31	34	29	28	38	18
Violence	29*	24	35*	15	22	7
Having meals together	58	56	60	53	56	49
Arguments	51*	46*	56*	34	30	38
Going out together	56	52	60	61	54	69
Watching TV	57	56	58*	43	46	40
Visiting relatives	57	52	61.5	59	64	53

*Significant difference from comparative school samples.

on the other hand the relatively high proportions including arguments and violence and the more mundane activity of watching TV suggest some degree of realism.

In terms of threats to family life, more of the young people considered that men concentrating too much on their work was damaging to family life than thought that women having a full-time job was. Unsurprisingly, more boys thought the latter and more girls thought the former but the only significant difference lay within the school sample where the proportion of boys considering that family life suffers because of women's full-time employment was double that of the girls. This was in line with the views of the young men in the Barnardo's study of young people's social attitudes (Roberts and Sachdev, 1996).

The component 2 questionnaire included a list of topics that might, or might not, have been covered in lessons at school or by parents and carers at home, one of which was 'family life'. About 25 per cent of those looked after claimed they had not been given any information about this from either source, more than in the school sample where 20 per cent said they had not been given information in school and 16.5 per cent said they had not been given any at home. The boys in public care were significantly more disadvantaged than their peers in the comparator group: 33 per cent as opposed to 14 per cent in the school sample said they not been given any information by parents or carers.

A subsequent question in the final section of the questionnaire specifically addressing education for parenthood – *Have you ever had any teaching about families or the relationships between members of the family?* – did not produce the same level of response, particularly in respect of the looked after sample. On this occasion, half of them reported that they had not received any instruction about families and family relationships. In the school sample just over one third claimed not to have had any, again many more than responded negatively to the first question.

Some variation in the level of response may be attributable to the fact that the first question was part of a long list where each topic was probably not given a great deal of individual consideration. The numbers responding to the two questions also varied slightly: in the school sample there were fewer responses to the second question (focused on teaching about family life) and in the looked after sample there were fewer responses to the question about information on family life having been given by parents or carers.

This question also asked respondents if they would like to have some teaching if they had not had any, or to have more if they had already received some. Just under one third of the looked after sample compared with only about one fifth of the school sample said that they would. But looked after young people, more than their peers who are not in public care, need to learn about family life and how family relationships function. Certainly their own experiences as related in interviews in both components suggest that in many cases the available parental role models were not ideal.

Parents

A major advantage of gathering data by both questionnaires and interviews is that the former provides the proportions that appear in certain categories while the latter helps us to understand what these mean. Thus the questionnaires administered in component 2 allowed us to gain basic information about contact and relationships with parents while the qualitative data from the interviews provided illustrative examples of the nature of these relationships and the young people's attitude towards their parents.

Since the existence of any relationship between young people in public care and their parents could not be assumed, this group was asked in the questionnaires how often they saw their parents. Overall there was much more contact with mothers than with fathers but variations in both the frequency of contact and the nature of the relationship were also observed according to the gender of the respondents (Table 2.2).

Just over half the respondents had no contact at all with their father; among the girls this rose to 60 per cent. Where contact did exist, just over one quarter of boys but only one fifth of girls said that they saw their father at least once a week. About a quarter of the sample had no contact with their mother, but, again, this was more often the case with girls (34

Table 2.2   Relationships with parents

	Looked after (%)			School (%)		
	Total	Male	Female	Total	Male	Female
Get on with mother:						
Very well	19	24.5	13	55*	60*	49*
Quite well	23	23	23	33	31	36
Neither well nor badly	22*	23*	21	9	7	11
Badly	6	7.5	4	2	–	4
Very badly	4	2	6	1	2	–
Do not see her at all	27*	21*	34*	–	–	–
Get on with father:						
Very well	15	21	9	38*	46*	28*
Quite well	12	15	9	35*	36*	35*
Neither well nor badly	11	13.5	9	15	10	22*
Badly	4	4	4	1	2	–
Very badly	5	2	7.5	1	–	2
Do not see him at all	52*	44*	60*	10	7	13

*Significant difference from comparative samples.

per cent) than with boys (21 per cent). However, of girls who did see their mother, more of them saw her on a daily basis than did boys, although the actual proportion having daily contact was very low (11 per cent). Nevertheless, boys were more likely than girls to see their mother weekly or even monthly and more likely than girls to spend weekends at their mother's home. The overall picture is that, apart from a handful of girls who had frequent and regular contact with their mother, the girls in public care saw their parents much less often than the boys did.

Relationships with mothers

Turning first to relationships with mothers for those in the looked after sample, we see that, while slightly more than one third of the girls claimed to get on either very well or quite well with their mother, this contrasted with almost half of the boys who described their relationship in this way (Table 2.2). Only a very low proportion (19 per cent) of respondents in the looked after sample claimed that they got on very well, and once again boys were more likely than girls to report this. The same pattern is visible in the school sample, with boys more frequently than girls (60 per cent as opposed to 49 per cent) reporting that they got on very well with their mother, but the proportions in the school sample are very much higher and the difference in respect of genders between them and the looked after sample is significant.

Overall 88 per cent in the school sample said they got on well or very well with their mother compared with 42 per cent in the looked after sample. Consequently in the looked after sample there were many more reports of either poor (10 per cent) or indifferent (22 per cent) relationships with mothers than in the comparator group where the proportions were, respectively, 3 and 9 per cent.

Inevitably, among the young people looked after the nature of the relationship with parents was governed by the reason for their being admitted to care. If they were there on a temporary basis and/or following a crisis which they did not perceive as involving rejection by the mother, then that relationship remained intact. One young woman, for example, repeated frequently throughout the interview that her mother loved her and that she would be returning to live with her once an impending court case was over.

> 'I love my family more than anybody and I just want to go home ... She (mother) loves me and everything, so. And I love my mum so that's it ... She's always considerate about me. She always cares about me and she's thinking about me all the time ... she tells me on the phone and that.' (Female)

A young man, being looked after following the death of his father and his mother's subsequent inability to cope, considered that she remained a commendable parent because, 'She's nice to us. She gives you respect.'

Such cases, however, were in the minority. Far more examples were given of relationships with mothers that were not satisfactory owing to rejection, neglect or abuse.

Among the school sample poor relationships with mothers hinged on relatively trivial (although no doubt significant to them) irritations such as mothers' nagging. Unlike the young people in the care sample, none reported relationships with mothers becoming difficult with the advent of a new partner. On the contrary, they were more likely to report a good relationship with the new partner.

Relationships with fathers

As we have already noted, nearly twice as many young people did not see their father as did not see their mother, with many more girls than boys having no contact. Moreover, the relationships with fathers that did exist were generally worse than those with mothers. Only 36 per cent of boys and 18 per cent of girls stated that they got on *either* very well *or* quite well with their father. While the proportion who claimed to have a poor relationship (9 per cent) was similar to the proportion reporting the same sort of relationship with their mother, far fewer reported getting on 'neither well nor badly' with their father than with their mother. But they often displayed an ambivalence in their attitude towards fathers, simultaneously rejecting them and trying to prove themselves to them:

> 'I don't want my life to go, you know, down the drain, and I want to show me dad. I want to say, "Look you fat bastard, I got on well without you. I did it on my own." Prove him wrong . . . I ain't seen him since I've been in care . . . I'm not interested in him no more.' (*Female*)

Although some boys recounted examples of little or difficult contact with fathers, the discrepancy between the genders in the quality and quantity of the relationships is noticeable. However, it is easier for fathers to maintain relationships with sons based on shared activities than it is for them to maintain relationships with daughters. Research on non-residential fathers after divorce shows that fathers are twice as likely to remain in contact with their children if they are all boys. While boys could be seen as 'mates and pals' girls were more apt to be kept at arm's length. (Simpson, McCarthy and Walker, 1995).

In the school sample, relationships between young people and their fathers were, similarly, not as good as those with mothers. Only 38 per cent claimed that the relationship was good compared with the 55 per cent who thought that the relationship with their mother was good, and this was more often the case for boys (46 per cent) than for girls (28 per cent). However, amalgamating the getting on 'very well' and 'quite well' categories shows proportions of 82 per cent for boys and 63 per cent for girls, significantly more than the proportions for either gender in the looked after sample quoted above. As with their relationship with mothers, the school sample girls were much more likely than the boys to report that they got on neither well nor badly with their father. In the looked after sample the difference between the genders in this respect was much smaller.

Although the proportion of young people who did not see their father at all was significantly lower in the school sample than in the looked after sample, again it was girls who were more likely to have no contact than boys (13 per cent as opposed to 7 per cent).

However, while young men in the school sample expressed a desire for an improved relationship with their father, in particular an ability to discuss sensitive and personal topics with him, young women, irrespective of their relationship with their mother, were more inclined to be indifferent. Those who complained in the interviews about the lack of time spent with parents because of the long hours that they worked, were more aggrieved by the time lost with mothers than with fathers.

Young people's perceptions of their parents

Qualitative data from the school sample suggested that parents' age was a major determinant of their relationship with their teenage children. Young parents were much more likely to be viewed in a favourable light than those described as 'old' (50 and over) who were described as 'too old to communicate with their kids'. In one group discussion in which two of the young people had parents of this age they made the following comments:

'They don't understand anything that's going on. They try but it just doesn't work.'

'Behind the times.'

'I think it's from the age they came from, because my mum and dad were brought up just after the war and they can still remember ration books – completely different!'

In one group a young woman referred to the fact that children of older parents tended to 'think you're an old fart and be embarrassed to be seen with you' whereas one of her peers in the group described with pleasure how her mother 'wears joggers and Reebock tops ... and she's really with it, all my friends really like her ... and she's really nice'.

In the qualitative part of component 2 many young people in public care indicated parental failure which frequently led them to believe that being in the care system was preferable to being at home. Such failings covered neglect, alcoholism, excessive strictness or what they perceived as inadequate parenting.

'(In more than a year) I've had a couple of letters off her (mother). I write. I've rung her once ... and that was on my birthday.' (*Female*)

'She rings me up but like I don't talk to her, because my mum's an alcoholic and every time she rings up she's always drunk, so I just put the phone down, I don't listen to what she says.' (*Female*)

'When I was younger my dad was really strict and I just went off the rails.' (*Female*)

'I'd rather be here than at home ... I wouldn't have done anything bad because it was just so strict there, like you couldn't do anything ... sometimes you think, "Oh, when I got to this age anyway I probably just go, like" because it was really *so* strict. I couldn't even go out and stuff like that, or ring up friends, and they couldn't even come, anything like that.' (*Female*)

'She was very negative towards me, and so obviously I'm negative towards myself ... I've deliberately tried to grow up much quicker basically because of my mum. She's very childish and I don't want to be like her.' (*Male*)

Although this young man made home visits on a regular basis these were not out of any desire to retain contact but rather to get away from the children's home where he was living:

'It's not particularly very good, it's just a break from here. Everywhere I go it's to escape from the other place.'

Interviews with these young people indicated that several girls had never had contact with their father and had never been given information about him, while others had experienced unsatisfactory relationships:

'Me mum and dad split up when I was seven. I lived with me mum until I were ten and then I went to go and live with me dad and then it didn't work out and everything, he was beating me up and stuff like that, over the slightest little thing. So I thought "Fuck it." Then I got social services involved so he chucked me out and then I went into care.' (*Female*)

Despite the fact that the looked after boys had better relationships with their fathers than looked after girls, nevertheless many of them had fathers who were not exemplary role models:

'I've not been treated well – my dad never cared, I don't even see me dad. I think I saw him once or twice since I've been in care.'

'I don't see my dad either because he gets violent. The last time I saw him was last summer. He got violent with me so I refused to see him ... I suppose if he was not violent then I would (see him), but at the moment I don't see it would be good if I did.'

'My dad's in prison so that don't say much.'

One 15-year-old young man described his entry into the care system and subsequent contact with his father:

'My mum died when I were four so I had to come into care. And my dad just kept getting pissed and that all the time so he said, "Right you little bastard, you're in care." So – fine ... He stabbed someone because they pushed me, so I told him and he went over and stabbed them. He got sent in prison for attempted murder ... He went in prison when I were going on five and he's just came out – so ... I stopped seeing him when I was 11 because I just didn't wanna know him then ... I've been seeing him the last couple of weeks because he lives where I go football training so I see him all the time ... but I was worried when he first moved over here again ... I thought he was going to do it again. He'll do it again and he'll get sent back in prison. He's just a mad bastard ... I ain't going to tell him when I get battered again!'

A major issue for these young people, and for the young mothers in component 1, was rejection of the young person by the mother in favour of a new partner. Girls were far more likely to be affected than boys but not exclusively so: one young man described the deterioration in the relationship with his mother following the arrival of her new partner in the following way:

'My mum? Well I don't really get on with her ...'
But you do go to see her, don't you? (*Researcher*)
'Yes I do. I've got a stepdad and all ... Sometimes I like him, sometimes I don't.'
Does he live with your mum? (*Researcher*)
Yes, unfortunately. He thinks he can boss me about but he can't.
How would it be if he wasn't there? (*Researcher*)
'Better, 'cos you'd have your own space and everything. 'Cos he's such a perfectionist. Everything's got to be done, like, how he wants it ... My mum used to be safe before she met him ... Like, she wouldn't tell us off as much. But now he's come, she's turned into a right old heap.'

One young woman offered the following description of her step-father's attitude towards her and the difficulties of home visits:

'He's a right knob-head ... He calls me a slapper and stuff like that so I call him names back and then it ends up in this big argument ... I end up walking out and I don't wanna phone her and she won't phone me so it just goes on for ages ... I would never put a boyfriend before me kids like she's done.'

The outcome of her experiences was a resolution not to treat her own children in the way that she had been treated by her mother. We might assume, therefore, that young people could learn from witnessing their parents' behaviour which had adversely affected them. However, without adequate knowledge of what a respectful relationship consists of or an alternative role model, it is questionable to what extent they are able to learn. This was illustrated by a young woman who described her mother's current relationship with a violent and alcoholic partner: she advocated hiding the visible nature of the relationship and the only lesson she was learning was toleration of violence for emotional reasons, neither of which was destined to increase a sense of self-worth.

> 'That's why she's got bruises on her. She wears skirts all the time. I've told her to wear trousers and she won't do that ... I tell my mum to leave him but she won't because she loves him. She loves him so much she can't leave.'

We learnt from the young mothers in component 1 that many of them felt that they had been rejected by their mothers in favour of a new partner and, though this may not have been the sole reason for their entering the care system, it was certainly seen as a contributory factor. When they became mothers the relationship with their own mother often changed again. Where mothers' new partners had been an original source of conflict, daughters were unlikely to change their attitude towards them but some, though by no means all, mothers became more prone to overriding the opposition of new partners in order to support their daughter and grandchild.

Mothers helped according to their ability; whether this was financial or with child care and support depended on their circumstances. One mother, who could not give monetary support and refused to babysit because she thought the children were unruly, nevertheless helped her daughter to find accommodation when she could not return home because of tensions with the mother's new partner, and she continued as the main source of help by visiting her every day. Many reported that their mother would be their first port of call in a crisis. Others turned to their mother for financial but not emotional help while for others the support came in emotional crises, over help with the baby or in practical ways when their mother's own precarious financial position precluded her giving money.

But for some young mothers the pattern of support was very different and involved a reversal of roles: having gained adult status by becoming a parent themselves, the young women were called upon to support their mother. This was frequently the case where the mothers were having marital problems or were in an abusive relationship with a new partner; ironically these relationships had often been a major factor in the young woman being looked after in the first place. Some responded by rejecting the mother who had rejected them:

'She only lives on the other side of the shops but she never comes round except when R (her new husband) hits her and she wants somewhere to stay. Now I've told her to stop coming because I don't want her problems.' (*17-year-old*)

But most of the 'older' mothers in the sample were willing, when required, to take on board their mother's problems along with their own, though it often meant they lost their own much-needed means of support:

'I can't really go to my mum with all the problems she's got.' (*18-year-old*)

'She doesn't really do a lot for me. I do just as much for her now as what she would do for me. I think she is probably more dependent on me now, it has sort of changed around now.' (*19-year-old*)

'I see my mum more or less every day. I try and meet her for dinner. Because my mum and dad's going through a divorce now so my mum's scared of being on her own ... My mum has actually stopped with us for four, maybe five, months because he can be a bit violent, my dad.' (*18-year-old*)

The caring role was not exclusive to those who had become mothers. In interviews in component 2 many young people in the looked after sample were able to cite occasions when they believed that, currently or in the past, they had been acting in an adult capacity. Such examples typically included caring for younger siblings, having to make a major decision or being the support for their peers with problems.

The questionnaire in component 2 included a set of questions on how young people viewed their parents' attitudes and behaviour towards them (Table 2.3). In the school sample nearly all parents were seen as helpful, caring and providing encouragement to do well at school. The majority also allowed young people to make their own decisions, allowed them to do the things they enjoyed and were willing to sort out problems at school or visit the school to talk to teachers. In response to all of these questions there was a difference according to gender, with the girls in the school sample viewing their parents as less supportive and more restrictive than the boys did. The girls more often felt they were ignored, treated like a baby and denied the things they enjoyed, and less often encouraged and supported at school. They also were less likely than boys to describe their parents as 'always' helpful and caring but more likely to describe them as 'usually' so.

The looked after sample displayed several areas of significant difference from the school sample. Overall the young people in the looked after sample did not experience the same level of support over the school-related issues as their non-looked after peers and their parents were seen as less helpful, caring and permissive than those of the school sample. There is a similar disparity according to gender as there is in the school sample, although the difference is especially marked in respect of girls feeling ignored by parents, being subject to parental control and not being encouraged to make decisions. This is supported by information gathered in interviews where many of the looked after young people, but especially the girls, reported that when they lived at home their parents had been very strict. Compared with the school sample girls, the looked after girls in the quantitative study fared significantly worse on all aspects with the exception of being treated like a baby.

Carers

However, it is important to bear in mind that it is carers, not parents, whose attitudes and behaviour towards them is more important on a daily basis. Consequently the questionnaire for the looked after sample contained an identical set of questions about carers (Table 2.4). Most of the sample thought that carers were helpful and encouraged them to do well at school and a substantial proportion thought they were also caring, let them do the things they enjoyed, liked them to make their own decisions and were willing to help with problems at school or visit the school. However, the young people felt that carers were inclined to treat them like a baby, take no notice of them and try to control what they did. A significantly greater proportion of boys than girls thought that carers ignored them, prevented them from doing the things they enjoyed and that they were not caring.

Overall carers were deemed to be more controlling than parents. On the other hand they were seen as more helpful and caring than parents, more likely to allow young people to do the things they enjoyed and to make their own decisions, and more willing to support and encourage them in their education. Girls appeared to believe that they had a better deal from carers than from their parents.

Further analysis of these questions was carried out to establish whether the same respondents replied negatively about carers *and* parents. The main areas where young people felt they suffered lay with having attention paid to them and having others control what they do. Of those replying to both questions, 25 per cent considered that both parents and carers always or usually took no notice of them and 43 per cent felt that parents and carers usually or always tried to control what they did. Thus a sizeable minority considered that their lives were controlled by others while little attention was paid to them.

It is important to remember that in this component of the study most of the young people being looked after were in residential care and that few responses to these questions were in respect of foster carers. The majority of them (and virtually all the girls) thought that their carers allowed them to do the things they enjoyed and most also thought that carers liked them to make their own decisions. The interviews in component 2 provided

Table 2.3   Description of parents' behaviour

	Looked after (%)			School (%)		
	Total	Male	Female	Total	Male	Female
They're very helpful:						
Always	40.5	51	30	49	62.5	33
Usually	47	40.5	54	48	33	64
Never	12	8	16*	3	4	2
They treat me like a baby:						
Always	17	14	21	13	7	19.5
Usually	19	17	21	30	33*	27
Never	64	69	58	57	60	54
They let me do the things I enjoy:						
Always	39	45.5	33	55*	74*	35
Usually	46	45.5*	47	40	21	60*
Never	14.5*	9	19*	5	5	5
They are caring:						
Always	58	65	50	69	76	61
Usually	31	30	32.4	28	20	37
Never	11	5	18*	3	4	2
They like me to make my own decisions:						
Always	44	50	38*	36	51	19.5
Usually	35	38	32	56*	42	71*
Never	21*	12	29*	8	7	10
They take no notice of me:						
Always	16	2	19*	17	23*	10
Usually	28	24	32	23	14	32.5
Never	56	67	48	60	63	57.5
They try to control what I do:						
Always	26	20	31	20	20	21
Usually	40	37	43	34.5	35	34
Never	34	43	26	45	45	45*
They encourage me to do well at school:						
Always	67	68	67	82*	89*	74
Usually	18	23.5*	12	16	9	24*
Never	15*	9	21*	2	2	2
If I have problems at school they are willing to help:						
Always	59	65	54	65	67	62.5
Usually	25	23.5	26	30	28	32.5
Never	16*	12	20*	5	4	5
They are willing to talk to teachers at school:						
Always	47	42	51	62*	70*	54
Usually	34	45.5*	23	31	24	39*
Never	19*	12	26*	7	6.5	7

*Significant difference from comparative samples.

Table 2.4   Description of carers' behaviour

	Looked after (%)		
	Total	Male	Female
They're very helpful:			
Always	48	44	51
Usually	50	54	47
Never	2	3	2
They treat me like a baby:			
Always	7	10	4
Usually	29	30	29
Never	63.5	60	67
They let me do the things I enjoy:			
Always	30.5	35	26
Usually	61	50	71*
Never	8.5	15*	2
They are caring:			
Always	54	45	62*
Usually	39	42	36
Never	7	13*	2
They like me to make my own decisions:			
Always	38	35	40
Usually	55	59.5	51
Never	7	5	9
They take no notice of me:			
Always	12.5	13	12
Usually	34	42*	26
Never	54	45	62*
They try to control what I do:			
Always	32.5	33	32
Usually	41	44	39
Never	26.5	23	29.5
They encourage me to do well at school:			
Always	82	82.5	82
Usually	15.5	15	16
Never	2	2.5	2
If I have problems at school they are willing to help:			
Always	71	65	77
Usually	21	24	19
Never	7.5	11	5
They are willing to talk to teachers at school:			
Always	66	58	73*
Usually	26	37*	16
Never	8.5	5	11

*Significant difference between males and females.

further corroboration of the freedom that young people might thus associate with living in residential care:

> 'Yes, cos, like, really they don't really care, sort of, because they're just there to look after you really, like, when you're inside there like, and that's it. Like, they'll give you money just to go out for the whole day . . . There is rules there but no one listens anyway and the staff don't care if you don't listen, so you don't listen.' (*Female*)

This was particularly apparent when compared with foster care, which many had experienced in the past. Although the young people initially claimed to prefer residential homes to foster care for this reason, they often subsequently revealed that they would appreciate a stricter routine. In a group discussion which began with the young people stating their preference for residential care because of the latitude it gave them, they went on to question among themselves whether this was unequivocally advantageous:

> 'I think there's more freedom in a children's home.'
> 'You can take advantage a bit more.'
> 'Coming in at whatever time you like, man.'
> 'More freedom and that.'
> 'We have a lot more choice over our lives without people telling us what to do all the time.'
> 'We can make our own choices.'
> 'That's a bad thing cos you've got no barriers, you've got no rules. No one saying "don't do this". It's just up to you.'
> 'There are rules, it's just that it's bad.'
> 'And if you break rules, you get in trouble and that but it's not big trouble.'

Two young people who had earlier in an interview described scenes of locking the care staff in rooms, staying out all night, pulling curtains down, setting off the fire alarm and generally 'running riot', as they described their activities, then went on to reflect:

> 'It (children's home) is better because you can stay out all night.'
> 'It depends. I mean, sometimes it can be good getting away with murder and other times it can't because I mean if you get away with too much . . .'
> 'You just keep on doing it again.'
> 'Yeah.'
> 'And again. And again and again.'
> **So would you like someone to stop you after a while?** (*Researcher*)
> 'Yes.'
> 'I've stopped now. I don't do owt wrong.'

Another, who had moved from residential into foster care, had likewise found that the excess of freedom could become tiresome and that once the novelty had evaporated she had been left wondering what to do next. Although she had found it difficult at first to adjust to living in foster care, she had subsequently found the presence of guidelines to be helpful.

In interviews with the looked after sample many young people themselves raised the topic of how they were treated by their carers and social workers. Those few who were living with foster carers and some of those in residential care spoke favourably of their carers' attitude towards them. In some instances all the care staff in a residential home were highly valued. In one group discussion respondents, who were otherwise highly critical of the care system, made the following point:

> 'But there's one good thing about this one (home) – you see, the staff, the staff are like very supportive and everything and if you have a problem and if you don't look too happy they approach you and ask you what's wrong and all that. And that's what I like about the staff here.'
> 'There's a good relationship.'
> 'Yes. You can talk to them in confidence and tell them anything.'

More often certain members of staff were singled out as favourites because they were prepared to listen, willing to invest additional effort into leisure activities or simply (in the case of young men) because they could talk about football.

But there is considerable variation in staff attitudes and in the ethos of residential homes (Berridge and Brodie, 1998) and some young people did not speak well of their experiences. Some found there was no one within the home to give them time or support and one young woman provided a graphic account of her unsuccessful attempts to have a confidential conversation with a member of staff.

> 'Brilliant example here last night. I came home from school and asked to speak to her (carer) in private and she goes "Okay". But first we have this little sort of meeting, but I was sitting there waiting for everyone to start talking and that, and then I couldn't stand it so I'd gone outside and then been pulled back in again. And then the meeting finishes, someone phones up and then she says, "I need to change the sheets . . . Will you come up and talk to me while I'm changing the bed then?" . . . And then someone else calls for me, and I've gone, "I'll be back in a minute". She's gone "Okay". I come back and she says, "I've just got to go and do . . ." so I come down, watching telly, and they've gone like "You can see her now", go into the office and she's standing there talking to N, and I've gone "Just forget it, okay", and she said "No, come on", so she walks into the TV room, the TV's on really loud and K's in there and it's about K I want to talk about, so obviously I don't want to talk while she's there. I'm like, "Can we go somewhere else?", and she said "No, we'll be all right", I said "I want to speak to you in private . . . You're not going to do this are you so we might as well forget it right now". I come upstairs

and gone back down, sat on the stairs and she goes, "Do you want a word with me?" I've gone, "Well, yes ..." and she said, "Yeah, but I asked you and you just ran off." I said, "Yeah because I wanted to speak to you in private but you weren't having any of it", and she goes, "Come on then" and then she takes me into the laundry room where there's a washing machine and a dryer ...'

Is it always like that if you want to have a private conversation? (*Researcher*)

'It is with this person. So I don't really speak to her very much, and she complains about it. Like she turned round to me and goes, "Why don't you speak to me?" And I says, "But you have to make a little time to listen to what I say to you, and then you're always round the little ones, you're more interested in what they're doing, you don't get talking to me, it goes in one ear and out the other so there's no point is there?". She goes, "I shall try harder then." Comes the next day she's doing exactly the same thing.'

A young man who felt particularly unsupported considered that the care staff did nothing to help him and the gender composition of the unit compounded the problems.

'It would be nice if it (help) actually came from here but ... they don't seem to ... sort of ... you could say identify more with you, especially me, I suppose I'm a little bit harder than the others and it takes a lot to identify with me, they say I'm difficult and that sort of thing, not in the way that I drink or do things I shouldn't do and that sort of thing, I'm not like that at all, total opposite ... They've actually said that I'm much different to the others and that they don't sort of know which way to guide me because of my personal issues. They're very ... just don't know what to do, so I suppose they do nothing at all really. That's the impression I get ... especially here, it's all female (staff).'

The position of care workers is difficult as they are frequently working under stressful circumstances which they are not always trained to meet. Many teenagers in residential care are very needy and expect a level of attention which cannot always be provided. In some cases a change in *their* attitude can produce a positive outcome, as this young woman, initially angry and disillusioned, discovered.

'But after a while the staff were brilliant. At first I used to shout my mouth off and swear at them, but, you know, I realised then that you need them more than they need you. They've still got a job whether you're doing what they tell you or not ... When I went in there ... I was just a no-hoper, dropped out of school, and you know. They taught me a lot, a lot of life skills, how to live and that. I think I wouldn't have turned out, settled down and that, the way I have if I hadn't have gone in there, and I wouldn't have had such a good relationship with my mum and dad.'

Despite some of the negative impressions given of carers, overall they were acknowledged as treating the young people better than their own parents did. Looked after respondents cited carers as people whom they trusted almost twice as often as they cited parents.

Many of the young people in the component 2 sample had previously been fostered and had experienced a breakdown in relationships with their foster carers: one young woman reported having had 16 different foster placements. Although several reported good experiences of foster care they tended to regard it as a temporary arrangement. As one young man remarked, 'I liked foster care. The only thing with foster care is you have to keep leaving'. They had been made well aware of the difficulties associated with being fostered when they were in their teens. Such experiences offer little in the way of positive reinforcement either about themselves or about successful relationships. One group made the following observations about foster care:

> 'It's really hard, innit, if you want to get teenage fostering.'
> 'The foster parents want younger children.'
> 'Well, with our generation there's more crime and everything, innit, and if you was fostered when you was young then it would be different circumstances if they want you or not?'
> 'They find it easier to look after younger children than people like us with all our problems.'
> **Is that how you see yourselves?** (*Researcher*)
> 'Yes, some us have got a lot of problems.'

Social workers

Social workers are the other significant adults in the lives of young people looked after and, along with carers, have the potential to demonstrate by example how to respect and interact with others. In component 1 many of the young mothers were highly critical of the unhelpful attitude and lack of support they received from their social workers (Corlyon and McGuire, 1997). Similar criticisms were voiced by many respondents in component 2. These young people, like those in component 1, found that lack of visits, broken appointments and frequent unavailability characterised their contact with social workers. For the young mothers in component 1, this was a two-edged sword because, although they felt rejected, they were also keen to escape their clutches for fear of social workers' involvement with the baby. Such considerations, however, did not apply to those in component 2 who merely experienced the rejection. A lively group discussion produced the following exchange about social workers:

'Well they don't do much for you anyhow.'

'Social workers are different.'

'They're not all the same, some are good, and some are not as good as others.'

Which ones are good ones? (*Researcher*)

'One you can have a good relationship with, somebody you can talk to, someone who'll help you.'

'It's not really the sex (of the social worker), it's if you can get on with them.'

'I don't get on with my social worker. My social worker's the worst.'

'They're stupid ... They won't come down and visit you, and they don't do much for you when they do come down.'

'When you do need things, they take about six months to get the things.'

'Well, that's care. That's social services, not the social worker.'

'It's the social worker's choice whether to come down.'

'Ah yes, but take this year, me and my social worker had a contract, innit. And my social worker's supposed to visit me every two weeks, like, every fortnight and I haven't ever seen my social worker. My social worker don't come round. She's too worthless ... she don't even phone.'

'They're full of shit.'

'Well my social worker's fine, I get on with her, and *she* helps me when I need help. And she's there if I need someone to talk to.'

'Most people expect the wrong things from social workers. They expect money and that but that's not what they're there for.'

'Well, you see, me and my mum's not getting on, yeah, and she sorts out all the contact and she expects me to go to my mum's house, but I can't go to my mum's house because my mum will chuck me out, you get me? So she don't do nothing for me. She don't phone me, and she don't come and see me, and she don't make contact and she don't do any planning for me. And she's supposed to be sorting out a family but she ain't done nothing about it.'

'You tell her in a meeting and she goes on about she gonna do it and she don't do it.'

'Mine is not reliable.'

'I've seen your social worker: she's a beast.'

'It's not what they look like.'

'(Mine is) easy to get on with and she'll listen to you and she'll help you. And you can have a mature conversation with her.'

'And you can have a laugh, as well.'

The view of the solitary young person in this group who felt that structural, not personal, issues were largely responsible, and that some of the blame rested on the unreasonable expectations of the young people themselves, echoed the views quoted earlier of the young woman in residential care who recognised that at least some responsibility for a good relationship with carers rested with herself. But this was not a common observation and most young people remained disappointed by the treatment they received from social workers.

Trust and respect from adults

An important aspect of relationships is the extent to which people feel that they are heard, respected, understood and trusted. Table 2.5 sets out the results of a question on this which was answered by the questionnaire respondents in component 2. Of those in public care, 57 per cent thought that carers listened to them, while only 36 per cent thought their parents did so. Similar proportions also considered that carers respected their ideas and understood them. In all of the responses from both samples, boys

Table 2.5   People understanding, trusting, listening to and respecting the ideas of young people

	Looked after (%)			School (%)		
	Total	Male	Female	Total	Male	Female
Respect my ideas:						
Parents	35	47	24	74*	80*	66*
Carers	55	59	51	–	–	–
Teachers	34	39	29	41.5	44	38
Siblings	42	47	37	38	41	34
Friends	70	67	73	71	71	70
Listen to me:						
Parents	36	45	28	74*	83*	62*
Carers	57	59	56	–	–	–
Teachers	45	47	44*	33	46	17
Siblings	49	55*	42	36	39	32
Friends	75	71	79	78	76	81
Understand me:						
Parents	34	46	24	61*	69.5*	51*
Carers	52	54	49	–	–	–
Teachers	32	40	26	28	39	15
Siblings	51*	56*	45	35	37	32
Friends	71	62	79	71	75	66
Trust me:						
Parents	41	53	29	74.5*	75*	74.5*
Carers	43	39	47	–	–	–
Teachers	38	35	41*	31	39	21
Siblings	50	55	45*	40	47.5	30
Friends	81	80	82	76	78	75.5

*Significant difference from comparative samples.

appeared to feel much better treated by their parents than girls did, though the differences between the genders were more marked in the looked after sample.

In interviews, some of the girls in the school sample complained about the dearth of time given to them by parents and this is an area where young people in public care might have scored more highly. They were not in the same situation as those young people who spent a great deal of time alone at home and whose parents were subsequently too exhausted to take notice of them. Nevertheless, many more parents in the school sample were deemed to respect the young people's ideas, trust, listen to and understand them than did carers in the looked after sample. And, as we have already noted, a substantial number of looked after young people felt that the main adults in their lives took no notice of them.

Unsurprisingly, significantly lower proportions of those in the looked after sample than in the school sample considered that their parents respected their ideas, listened to them, trusted and respected them. They were more inclined to think that carers fulfilled these tasks to a much greater extent than their parents, with the exception of being trusted. Fewer of them felt that carers trusted them and this was especially the case for boys, who were more inclined to feel trusted by parents than carers.

When asked how many people they could trust, more respondents in the school sample than in the looked after sample replied that there was no-one, although the numbers are too small to attach significance to them. Those in the looked after sample were more inclined to place their trust in one or two people (44 per cent of the looked after sample compared with 27 per cent of the school sample) whereas those in the school sample typically felt they had a wider circle of people who could be trusted: 38 per cent, compared with 29 per cent of the looked after sample, felt they could trust three or four people. In the list of people whom they thought they could trust, 91 per cent of the school sample compared with 37 per cent of the looked after sample cited parents and/or family.

As we have observed, social workers were seen neither as offering trust nor as worthy of receiving it. Only four of the 106 questionnaire respondents cited them in the list of people they could trust. Most of the young people sensed that they were not valued in their own right by social workers and that their feelings and views were not respected. One young mother made the following comment:

'Some of them like K sit there and tell you what's right. They don't listen to your point of view as well, they don't say, "Well do you think you should be doing this? Do you think this is right?" They say, "This is right, this is what you should be doing." They don't listen.' (*17-year-old with baby, aged five months*)

In a discussion about the nature of trust, one young woman in component 2 compared the trust lost when a relationship ended because of betrayal as 'like having a social worker. They've said a lot of things to you, and then done another', to which a young man in the group added, 'I hate it when people do things behind your back and don't tell you the truth afterwards'.

Not only was trust lacking in the social worker relationship but so, too, was respect. One young woman, whose account was not unusual, reported that her social worker was extremely difficult to contact and did not respond to messages left for her but would then telephone her at school during lessons.

> '... you ring up and they say, "Can I take your number?" and she knows what time I get in and everything, so she phones up ten minutes before ... and she'll say, "Can you get B to phone me". You phone her and she's out, "Okay then", so she phones you up in the middle of your lesson, your favourite lesson, so you get called over ..., she's got this thing about phoning me up in my favourite lessons, like English, most English lessons I'll get called out ... Usually it's next to dinner time, so you get dragged out of school at dinner time.'

Summary points

While the perceptions of family life held by the two samples in component 2 overlapped on some items, a significantly higher proportion of young people in the looked after sample than in the school sample cited both violence and arguments. Within the looked after group, girls were more likely than boys to mention these.

Looked after young people were much more likely than the school sample young people to report that they had not received any teaching at school or information in their home setting about family life, and boys appeared to be more disadvantaged than girls in this respect. Nearly one third of looked after young people said that would like some teaching on the topic.

Many of the looked after young people in component 2 had parents who were not ideal role models. For the young mothers in component 1 this often posed particular problems in respect of their own parenting skills. In addition, once they had achieved adult status by becoming parents, they were often seen by their own mothers as a source of support in their own troubled lives.

Half the looked after young people in the component 2 sample had no contact with their father and a quarter had no contact with their mother. Relationships with parents that did exist were much worse than those experienced by the young people in the school sample; girls in particular appeared to suffer in this respect.

Although carers were able to compensate to some extent, especially in providing support over school-related problems, nevertheless the combined effect of parents' and carers' attitudes and behaviour was not comparable to that of school sample parents. A not inconsiderable proportion of looked after young people felt that they were simultaneously ignored and controlled by both parents and carers.

Some young people reported a high level of support from carers but this was not uniform across the component 2 sample and there existed examples of young people who felt that carers showed no interest in them.

Social workers were viewed by most looked after young people in both components as generally unhelpful, untrustworthy and unavailable. In times of crisis they were unreliable and unresponsive.

Trust and respect appeared to be the main ingredients missing in the relationships that the looked after young people had with the significant adults in their lives. Even though many young people in public care felt that they were treated well by their carers and a quarter cited them as people they would trust, their level of trust contrasted significantly with that which the teenagers in the school sample felt they gained from or could give to their parents or other family members.

3 Relationships with peers

Given the poor relationship which young people in public care often experience with adults we explored the extent to which their relationships with peers might offer some compensation. This includes opposite-sex relationships which other researchers have indicated are particularly important for those with difficult family relationships (Pawlby, Mills and Quinton, 1997).

Siblings

In the component 2 samples, the young people in public care tended to have more siblings than those in the comparator group. For the former the average number of brothers was 2.35 and of sisters 2.09 while for the school sample the averages were 1.49 and 1.24 respectively. The looked after sample also had more complex family arrangements which included children from parents' former and new relationships.

Their brothers and sisters appeared to play a more significant role in their lives than did the siblings of many of the young people in the school sample. In terms of understanding and trusting them, listening to them and respecting their ideas, the young people looked after were much more likely to attribute these characteristics to their siblings than to their parents (see Table 2.5). The boys were far more inclined to do so than the girls. The level of support they appeared to receive from their brothers and sisters was greater than that which the young people in the school sample appeared to have: for the boys the main areas of significant difference lay in the greater extent to which they felt listened to and understood by their siblings while the for the girls the major difference was that they thought their siblings trusted them.

Friends

Relationships with friends are especially important for this age group, irrespective of their domestic circumstances or living arrangements. Respondents to the questionnaire in component 2 were asked whether they had a special friend to whom they could talk about personal things.

Several young people felt the need to respond in a way that indicated that this was of no concern to anyone else (some more politely than others), which itself is interesting since many of the other questions that they answered were potentially more intrusive. Perhaps this indicates a protective attitude towards friendships and certainly the results from those who did reply point to the importance of friendships for both samples. Overall there was no difference between the samples (Table 3.1) with the majority, and especially the girls, claiming they had a special friend. However, among the boys as many as 31 per cent in the looked after sample and 27 per cent of those in the school sample said they did not.

Friends were most often cited by both samples in the list of people whom they thought they could trust. In addition, as we saw in Table 2.5, friends were seen by the young people as more likely than parents, carers, teachers or siblings to be the ones to trust them, listen to them and understand them, but they were particularly important to young people in public care in these respects. The young people in public care also, unlike the young people in the school sample, considered friends to be the main source of respect for their ideas.

However, many young mothers in component 1 of the sample reported difficulty in making and retaining friendships, either because they did not trust others or because their experiences of moving placements had made it hard for them to keep in touch with friends. Some had low self-esteem which made them unsure about the nature of friendship.

'I haven't really got any close friends since I left school and that, I just forget about them. And they're really bitchy anyhow so I'd be better off on my own ... I just keep everything to myself.' (*16-year-old*)

'I don't go out to meet new friends, so I've not really got any close friends ... I mean, when I take her (daughter) to school I talk to the mums there, but I wouldn't ever dream of saying, "Oh, come back for a coffee." Because that's not me, I just wouldn't do that. Or if they said, "Come back for a coffee" I'd probably say, "No, you're all right, I've got to go home." I don't know, I panic because I know I'm going to be on my own in someone's house and I don't know them.' (*18-year-old*)

Table 3.1   Percentage of respondents who have a special friend they can talk to about personal things

	Looked after			School		
	Total	Male	Female	Total	Male	Female
Special friend	82	69	94	82	73	93

Some, however, managed to maintain friendships, and friends were a valued contact, albeit not usually a means of support. They were there primarily for leisure and relaxation times and in one case for protection.

'I've got friends and I've picked up some from children's homes and I still keep in contact with them. Some of them are really good friends.' (*16-year-old*)

'Mine are mostly black that I've grown up with and they're there if I get into fights and things like that.' (*16-year-old*)

Amongst the young mothers in the Thomas Coram study (Phoenix, 1991) a majority neither confided in others nor could see the value in doing so. Sometimes their reluctance to share confidences with friends was occasioned by anxiety either that confidentiality would not be maintained or that the nature of the relationship would be changed in such a way that friends would then take advantage of them. Biehal and others (1995) point to a correlation between poor relationships with parents and poor friendship networks. The absence of trust in the former makes it difficult for young people to have faith in friends. They also refer to the ability of other young people to prey on vulnerable care leavers who, out of insecurity and loneliness, allow themselves to be dominated by the unreasonable demands of friends resulting in even more physical and emotional chaos in their lives. In component 1 of our study, several of the young mothers described how friends who were homeless or unsatisfactorily housed had taken advantage of their more comfortable living arrangements and in some cases had caused damage which had necessitated their being re-housed.

Opposite-sex relationships

According to data published in 1994, the median age for first sexual intercourse was 17 years for young people in the 16–24 years age group, although nearly one fifth of women and one quarter of the men in this age group had their first experience of sexual intercourse before the age of 16 (Wellings and others, 1994). But data from the Health Education Monitoring Survey of 1995 (Health Education Authority, 1996) indicate that the average age of first intercourse for 16–19-year-olds was 15.2 years for men and 15.5 years for women, suggesting a constant decrease in age.

Religious affiliation is one factor that appears to delay first sexual activity while peer influences, pressure from partners, previous sexual abuse and the presence in the family of an older sexually active sibling are likely to advance it. Sexual activity increases as socioeconomic status decreases and low socioeconomic status is also closely related to low levels of academic achievement and interest. Exclusion or suspension from school, drug and alcohol use, smoking, violence and theft are considered by some researchers to represent a 'package' of behaviours or a certain lifestyle to which adolescent sex and pregnancy are linked (NHS Centre for Reviews and Dissemination, 1997).

Many of the young people in our study who were looked after had some of the above characteristics. Few had involvement in any religion: only 18 per cent of the looked after sample compared with 26 per cent of the school sample said they were either religious or very religious. Furthermore, although it would be simplistic to claim that, lacking trust and respect, all looked after young people turn towards sexual relationships in an attempt to feel valued, it would be equally naive to assume that there was no connection.

The teenagers, predominantly aged 14–15, in component 2 were asked on the questionnaire whether they currently had a boy or girlfriend and whether they had had one in the past. The questions did not specify whether this was a sexual relationship. In the school sample 34 per cent claimed to have a current relationship while 83 per cent claimed to have had such a relationship in the past. In the looked after sample the proportions were higher at 55 and 96 per cent respectively. In both samples a higher proportion of boys than girls stated that they were currently in a relationship, with the looked after boys especially likely to claim that they were (61 per cent as opposed to 38 per cent of the school sample).

Most of the young mothers and pregnant young women in component 1 claimed to have had their first sexual intercourse around the age of 14 or 15, some even earlier. While not necessarily advocating this as an appropriate age to embark on a sexual career, they did not feel constrained to hide the fact that they had done so. However, they did not favour sex at the age of 12 or 13: their concerns lay around the stage of physical development rather than issues of morality or legality. They did uniformly see having a boyfriend as the norm among young people in public care. One 15-year-old mother in component 1 whose social worker identified the current lack of boyfriend as the young woman's major source of concern commented, 'People in care, they've always got a boyfriend'. Another young mother offered an explanation:

> 'Because people in care have such a shitty life they feel better if they're going to bed with someone. They get to feel that "they love me because they sleep with me" but their past has a lot to do with it.' (*15-year-old*)

The aim of the questions on opposite-sex relationships in the quantitative part of component 2 was to explore attitudes rather than behaviour and consequently most questions were focused in a more general way. Among the young people in the school sample 81 per cent agreed with the statement that 'young people have sex too early' compared with 69 per cent in the care sample (Table A.1, Appendix B). The boys in public care were least likely to think that this was true.

Nevertheless, the responses to other questions showed a high level of acceptance of sexual relationships under the age of 16.

In the series of vignettes about a 15-year-old couple, respondents were asked to decide whether the couple should have a sexual relationship. There was very little difference between the samples in the nature of the responses (see Table A.2, Appendix B): the majority favoured going ahead provided both agreed and they used contraception. Boys, but especially those looked after, were more inclined to advocate this than girls in either sample. Young people who themselves had a boyfriend or girlfriend were more likely than those without to indicate that the couple should have a sexual relationship. In the care sample this was especially so for the girls.

Notwithstanding these responses most young people (both genders in both samples) thought that the age at which it was 'all right' for young people to begin having sex was 16 (Tables 3.2 and 3.3). This might owe more to an awareness of the legal position than to their beliefs, although about a quarter of the young people in public care and a third of those in the comparator sample appeared not to realise that sex between boys and girls under 16 was against the law (Table 3.4).

Few thought that older than 16 was an appropriate age while a substantial proportion thought that younger than 16 was. A greater proportion of the boys in public care than the girls considered that sex under the age of 16 was all right for both boys and girls, but more boys than girls favoured 14 as opposed to 15. In the looked after sample both boys and girls thought that under 16 was equally appropriate for both genders but the school sample boys apparently operated a double standard, believing that it was all right for boys to start having sex at a lower age than it was for girls. Interestingly, the school sample girls were much more likely than the girls who were looked after to advocate ages under 16 and they did so for both genders.

A subsequent set of questions asked respondents' views about sexual activity under the age of 16. The responses to these questions, set out in Table 3.4, did not always accord with their responses to the questions

Table 3.2 Age at which it's all right for girls to start having sex

	Looked after (%)			School (%)		
Age	Total	Male	Female	Total	Male	Female
14	17	21*	12	9	10	11.5
15	15	15	15	18	17.5	27*
16	45	37.5	54*	42	57.5*	35
17	4.5	4	5	5	5	8
18	13.5	15	12	12	10	19
Mean	15.7	15.5	16	15.95	15.9	16
Mode	16	16	16	16	16	16

*Significant difference from comparative samples.
Columns do not total 100 per cent: some values were below 14 and over 18 years.

Table 3.3   Age at which it's all right for boys to start having sex

	Looked after (%)			School (%)		
Age	Total	Male	Female	Total	Male	Female
14	16	21	10	16	18	14
15	16	12.5	20	22	18	28
16	41	35	47.5*	36	41	28
17	7	6	7.5	3	4.5	21
18	12.5	15	10	14	9	0
Mean	15.7	15.5	15.9	15.9	15.5	16.4
Mode	16	16	16	16	16	15/16

*Significant difference from comparative samples.
Columns do not total 100 per cent: some values were below 14 and over 18 years.

Table 3.4   Thinking about people under 16 do you agree that sexual intercourse is ...

	Looked after (%)			School (%)		
	Total	Male	Female	Total	Male	Female
Fine in a steady relationship	80	90*	69	72	62	82
Fine if both agree	75	81	70	81	84	78
Fine if you use protection against pregnancy	80	89	71	79	75.5	82
Fine if you use protection against sexually transmitted diseases	78	85	72	77	78	76
Against the law	77	85*	68	64	52	76
Something parents and carers would disapprove of	72.5	78	68	70	67	73
More likely if you've been drinking alcohol	54	46	63	63	67*	58
OK, everybody does it	36	39	33	31.5	35	27
One way to keep your boy/girlfriend	13	13	12	18	25*	9

*Significant difference from comparative samples.

above. Roughly equal proportions (ranging between 70 and 80 per cent) in both samples agreed that sexual intercourse under the age of 16 was 'fine' in a steady relationship, if both partners agreed, and if protection was used against pregnancy and against sexually transmitted diseases. This is a much greater proportion supporting under-age sexual activity than was shown in responses to the earlier question. Once again, more boys than girls in public care agreed that it was fine in a steady relationship and if protection was used against pregnancy, while the gender position was reversed in the school sample.

Similar proportions in both samples also agreed that parents and carers would disapprove (around 70 per cent), with more boys than girls believing this to be the case in the looked after sample but the reverse being the case in the school sample. More looked after young people than school sample young people agreed that it was 'OK because everybody does it' (36 versus 31.5 per cent) and boys were more inclined than girls to agree. Fifty-four per cent as opposed to 63 per cent in the school sample agreed that it was more likely after drinking alcohol, and looked after girls and school sample boys were most aware of a link with alcohol consumption. Overall very few respondents considered it was a way to keep a boyfriend or girlfriend but more in the school sample (18 per cent) than in the looked after sample did so (13 per cent) and the highest proportion was noted in the boys in the school sample (one quarter).

Pressure

Despite some ambiguities in responses, it seemed that young people were generally accepting of early sexual activity. We therefore explored whether respondents considered that young men and young women felt under pressure to have a boyfriend or girlfriend and, if so, where such pressure came from (Tables 3.5 and 3.6).

Overall the main source of pressure was from friends of their own age and sex but the boys in public care thought that boys were much less susceptible to this than the school sample boys did. In response to a previous question the boys in the school sample proved to be much more likely than those in the looked after sample to believe that their friends made them feel that sex was the most important thing in a relationship (58 per cent compared with 38 per cent).

Looked after young people were far *less* likely to be susceptible to the media and to magazines than the school sample, especially in respect of

Table 3.5   Pressure on girls to have a boyfriend

Main sources of pressure	Looked after (%)			School (%)		
	Total (n = 44)	Male (n = 21)	Female (n = 23)	Total (n = 53)	Male (n = 25)	Female (n = 28)
Friends of own age and sex	37	18	19	45	21	24
Boyfriends	31*	13	18*	19	10	9
Class-mates	28	13	15	36	16	20
Siblings	10	5	5	14	10	4
Media	15	9	6	34*	19*	15*
Magazines	22	11	11	35	17	18

*Significant difference from comparative samples.
Values are numbers of respondents.

Table 3.6   Pressure on boys to have a girlfriend

Main sources of pressure	Looked after (%)			School (%)		
	Total (n = 39)	Male (n = 13)	Female (n = 26)	Total (n = 52)	Male (n = 26)	Female (n = 26)
Friends of own age and sex	33	10	23	47	23	24
Girlfriends	20	7	13*	13	9	4
Class-mates	26	7	19	39	18*	21
Siblings	16	3	13	24	15*	9
Media	15	4	11	23	14*	9
Magazines	19	5	14	25	14*	11

*Significant difference from comparative samples.
Values are numbers of respondents.

pressure on girls to have a boyfriend. On the other hand, the looked after young people, of both genders, were much more likely than those in the school sample to think that pressure came from partners. Nearly as many looked after girls thought that pressure on girls came from boyfriends as thought it came from their own friends, which was not the case in the school sample. But looked after boys, too, believed that girls were subject to pressure from boyfriends, and to a far greater extent than did their peers who were not looked after. It is particularly noteworthy that a much higher proportion (of both genders) in the looked after sample thought that girlfriends put pressure on boys, and the difference between the girls in the two samples was significant.

The interviews in component 1 had earlier explored whether in general there is pressure for young people to have a boy or girlfriend and whether there is then pressure to have sex with them. It emerged that, at a relatively early age, a relationship of some sort with a member of the opposite sex was frequently essential if young people in public care were to avoid feeling left out and were to be accepted within a certain group.

'There's group pressure ... You either pair off or you're gooseberries! I don't know, it's not just from your friends that you hang around with, it's, say, from your school, you're either a goodie two shoes or you're in with the gang! To be in the gang you've got to be bad, type of image.' (*18-year-old*)

Many young women considered that there was pressure to engage in sexual activity which arose from two main sources: the boyfriend and the peer group and, sometimes, an overlapping of the two. Group pressure seemed less easy to deal with than pressure from boyfriends. It was also more complex because it could come from different sources: from friends of the same gender, from a group consisting of couples or from the group to which the boyfriend belonged. Many considered this to play an important role in adolescent life:

'I think in everywhere you'll get certain girls where they'll be a lot more mature and they'll have older boyfriends and they will sleep with them. So – the people around them, they know they've got boyfriends and they're not sleeping with them and it's like, "What, you haven't slept with him yet?" And the guys, it's like, "You've been going out with her so long, why haven't you given her one yet?"' (*18-year-old*)

'... if you're knocking about with a group of girls and none of them have got boyfriends, it just doesn't really come in to it ... But when you're in with the popular ones they've all got boyfriends and that's all that's ever talked about: "I've done it with him and I've done it with him" and "Have you done it?" You can't say no because you feel a right mug then, don't you?' (*18-year-old*)

Boys, it was felt, had a certain macho image to maintain, not only to satisfy their own view of themselves but also to meet the requirements of their own peer group.

'All you heard was, "Yeah, she's nice ain't she? Oh I'm going to get her.' (*16-year-old*)

'The lads, the unpopular ones, think they're just, like, the nobodies in school so they don't have anything to live up to. But the popular ones have, like, standards to live up to.' (*18-year-old*)

This could be translated into additional pressure on the young woman if she cared for her boyfriend and cared about his reputation in his peer group, rendering resistance to the plea of 'Come on, I've got to go and tell my mates that we've been together', as reported by one 18-year-old, very difficult.

For young women who had been the victims of abuse, of which there was a not insignificant number in this small sample, the problems of pressure were sometimes more subtle. One young woman articulated them thus:

'Like I said with the problems I have had, I was also abused by my brother [as well as her father] when I was younger. I mean, obviously I didn't like it but it makes you think you do like it because that is getting you aroused as it does. And I think maybe if that didn't happen, if I hadn't gone through it, I wouldn't have been doing what I was doing so early.' (*19-year-old*)

The remarks of many of the young women quoted above might be equally applicable to the general population but for those looked after, and especially those in residential care, there was a particular pressure to engage in sexual activity:

'I think there was more in the home because everyone else was (having sex) and as someone in there you feel left out so you do it for the fact that everyone else does it ... He didn't pressure me into having sex with him but it was purely the fact that M had someone, T had someone, F had someone and if you are left out you've got no one.' (*18-year-old*)

Living in residential care also brought unique opportunities:

'But in a children's home anyway they must know. I mean, if you are at home and you have got a boyfriend your parents are there to keep an eye on you but if you are in a children's home and the staff arc just there they don't know what goes on when they go to bed at night.' (*19-year-old, previously living in a children's home*)

'They just let you get on with it really. It's nowt to do with them really. They don't really interfere with owt like that.' (*18-year-old, previously in an independent living unit*)

'They never knew nothing about me. They never knew whether I was in or out, or where I was going or what time I'd be back ... because I didn't want them to know.' (*16-year-old, previously living in a children's home*)

When she became pregnant at the age of 15, this young woman was, theoretically, living in residential care with a care order in effect but in reality was living with friends. She returned to the home only for food, clean clothes and a bath.

One young woman's experience of living in a residential school was that there were always discussions among the residents about 'who was going out with who.' She was aware that the staff knew what was happening and made some attempt to stop it. 'They say things like "Yous (*sic*) are too young, you want to find your own way before you get involved in relationships with other people."' But when she became involved with the boyfriend who later became the father of her child she was approaching 16 and 'once you're 16 they cannot really say owt.' No attempt was made to separate them, and they were not only left in peace to pursue the relationship but were always treated as a couple by the staff.

However, one young woman in component 2 who had been placed in residential care with little female company had formed friendships with the boys only to find that she was under close supervision from the staff who suspected (incorrectly) that she was having a sexual relationship. This was, she pointed out, forbidden in children's homes.

'... I got on well with the lads and some of the staff got the wrong idea – like a girl hanging round with a bunch of lads. But I did it because the one girl was pregnant so she didn't get out much; and the other one was just crazy, she'd just go anywhere on her own. So I hung round with the lads and you're not allowed to have relationships in homes with a boy ... They're really strict on that – which is fair enough, cos when you're living under the same roof you can get up to all sorts, can't you? They can't really stop you, but if they suspect that you are then they keep a close eye on you and try and keep you apart.'

Local authority policy and practice

In the component 1 discussions with local authority staff, it emerged that sexual relationships between young people looked after were seen as a particularly problematical area but were without a recognised policy framework. With no overt policy to turn to, replies tended to come in the form of 'normal practice' and this appeared in turn to address each case individually. Thus considerations were given to whether there was any actual or potential coercion, no matter how subtle, and whether there was a significant age difference between the young people concerned. One interviewee remarked that this was a difficult area because young women being looked after had a tendency to form relationships with 'older men' by which was meant young men in their late teens or early twenties. In such cases the older partner might be deemed to be exerting undue pressure on the younger one, although in reality this may not be so. Another respondent reported that the fathers of the babies of young women who were under 16 were themselves usually 'a product of the care system'. This is not surprising as young people with similar adverse experiences tend to associate with one another (Quinton and others, 1993).

In two authorities a generally strict approach was taken towards this issue, and partners living in the same residential unit were always separated. Both authorities reported a low rate of teenage pregnancy amongst those being looked after. In one of these, however, the rate of pregnancy amongst young women who had recently ceased to be looked after was reported to be high (13 per cent of care leavers), suggesting that the effectiveness of such intervention is short lived.

No respondent was aware of a specific policy relating to sexual activity involving a minor. Again, each case was considered on an individual basis. Although they stated that there was considerable leeway on prosecutions, the general view was that if there was coercion *or* if there was a large age difference between the parties then prosecution was likely to be considered.

In some cases the lack of policy was reported to be a positive choice to counteract 'non-progressive attitudes' which might be encountered in some members of policy-making committees. A stated policy would leave little room for manoeuvre in a case, for example, where separation and, possibly, prosecution might not be in a young person's best interests. One respondent commented that 'In the past there have been some fairly positive and creative practice-based efforts to deal with these situations when they arose but that is happening outside the remit of policy.' Another reported that in that particular area of the country under-age sex was a very common occurrence in the wider community and it was, therefore, difficult to discriminate where young people in public care were concerned.

The difficulties of combining a hard-line policy with a child-centred approach are apparent. An inflexible procedure will, for example, contradict a policy document stating that 'If there is a conflict of interest between an adult and a child and in all decisions relating to their future, the child's interests must be given first consideration and their voice must be heard.' A similar situation would arise with policies on the recording of confidential information, which appeared also to be absent. One respondent, in pointing out the disadvantages of any policy – 'Our problem is that if there was a written guideline it would be a very uncompromising and unforgiving one' – indicated that in its absence there were examples of staff taking a 'very level-headed, panic-free' view which allowed them to 'try and influence what happens positively'.

Carers themselves, lacking policy and guidance, were often in a difficult position on this matter. In response to a question about policy on sexual activity one experienced carer replied:

> 'I don't know if there's an actual policy but certainly we would treat each individual case on its own merits, I suppose. I mean, there's a policy that staff go through training for ... we do have training courses.' (*Residential carer*)

For workers in independent living units the position is somewhat different in that they are dealing only with young people aged 16–18 years. Although rules about not having live-in partners exist and are maintained, discussions about current sexual activity can be open, particularly where workers have a good relationship with residents. In some cases this can give them privileged information, albeit with some of the characteristics associated with exaggeration and bravado:

> 'We have sessions on safe sex and pregnancy and I'm all for it because I've known girls meet somebody and within half an hour of meeting them they're in bed with them ... I was sat here one night with three girls ... and we were chatting and then the conversation was "Where have you had sex?". "In the lift." And one of the girls, some time ago, by the time she got to the nineteenth floor it was over! Security had it on tape ... And it was "On the stairs, on the market stalls, subways, outside the block, car parks..."' (*Residential carer*)

Likewise in mother and baby units where rules prohibiting overnight visitors exist there could still be a more relaxed attitude towards sexual matters. A social worker described her visit to a 15-year-old mother living in such a unit and her introduction to a new boyfriend:

> 'No, I don't know him. I met him the other week. I went up to see her and he was lying in her bed. I said, "Has he stayed?" She said, "No." I

said, "Is he supposed to be lying in your bed?" and she said, "Well what can they do?" I said, "What *can* they do? That's right." I just chatted to her with this young man lying in bed fast asleep ... he grunted a few times and said hello. I said, "Have you had a hard night?" He was only about 15 or 16 himself. But she wasn't at all embarrassed or anything about it, just carried on. Not at all bothered, didn't care what I thought.' (*Social worker*)

Summary points

Relationships with friends had paramount importance for young people in both samples of component 2 in terms of listening, trusting, understanding them and respecting their ideas. But the greater exploration of friendships in component 1 suggested that looked after young people experience difficulty in sustaining long-term friendships and are more likely to rely on friends for leisure and diversionary activities than for emotional support.

Siblings were considered to be significantly more reliable as a source of understanding for the looked after young people than they were for those in the school sample. Looked after girls also thought that their siblings trusted them more than many other people did, while the boys thought that they listened to them more.

As regards opposite-sex relations, our findings imply that young people have a high level of acceptability of sexual intercourse under the age of 16 if it is both safe and consensual. Looked after boys were most aware of the legal position and of an anticipated high level of parental or carer disapproval but were still more inclined to believe it acceptable because it was commonplace. However, young people who are looked after do not appear to engage in sexual activity as a means of maintaining a relationship.

The lack of interest and respect shown by adults to many looked after young people might be one reason why they appeared to attach significance to having a sexual relationship, thereby feeling special to someone, at a relatively early age. They also apparently experienced considerable pressure to have a partner, primarily from friends of their own age and sex, and in that respect they were fairly similar to their peers who were not looked after. Where they differed, however, was in pressure from the opposite sex: both girls *and* boys in the looked after sample agreed that there was substantial pressure from the opposite sex to have a girl or boyfriend, which was not a view shared by the school sample. For those living in residential care there is additional pressure to conform to 'standard' behaviour (being involved in a sexual relationship) for fear of being excluded or marginalised, while at the same time there is enhanced opportunity to do so because of the limits of close supervision.

4   Information about relationships, sex and contraception

If, as we have indicated, young people are under considerable pressure to embark on sexual relationships at a relatively young age, how prepared are they for doing so? This chapter addresses the extent to which young people in public care are given adequate and appropriate information about sex and relationships which would allow them to make informed decisions about whether or when to engage in sexual relationships. Comparisons are made with the young people from the comparator group in component 2.

Inadequate sex education is consistently emphasised in explanations for the relatively high rate of teenage pregnancy in Britain (NHS Centre for Reviews and Dissemination, 1997). In other countries where sex education is treated more openly, notably Sweden, Denmark and the Netherlands, fewer teenagers become pregnant (Grunseit and Kippax, 1994). The issue for looked after young people is whether they have the same access to sex and relationship education, however limited, as their peers who are not looked after receive.

Sex education: policy and practice

Sex education in school

Under Section 241 of the Education Act 1993 sex education is now compulsory in maintained secondary schools in England and Wales. Parents, or those with legal responsibility for children, have the right to withdraw their children from any lessons about sex which are not part of the National Curriculum. Before the recent legislation school sex education was not of a uniform standard throughout England and Wales (Thomson and Scott, 1992) nor were its content and style necessarily of a standard that met the needs of its audience. It tended to be focused on sex and the negative outcomes (disease and unintended pregnancy) of sexual activity and ignored issues around relationships and feelings. Department for Education and Employment guidance now stresses that sex education should cover more than the reproductive system. Ideally, and to meet the wishes of parents and young people (Hirst, 1994), it should address a wider range of issues which might include abortion, abuse, relationships and the life choices other than motherhood that are available to young women.

A key issue for the looked after population, however, is that they experience more periods of absence or exclusion from school than their peers who are not being looked after. A Social Service Inspectorate report demonstrated that 12 per cent of school-age children did not attend school regularly or were excluded. This proportion rose to 25 per cent at Key Stage 4 (Department of Health, 1995a). Thus they are more likely to miss the sex education, however limited, that is available.

Local authorities' policies and practices

The Guidance and Regulations accompanying the Children Act 1989 sets out the duties of agencies who are looking after children in respect of their education about sex and contraception:

> The experience of being cared for should also include the sexual education of the young person. This may, of course, be provided by the young person's school, but if it is not, the SSD or other caring agency responsible for the young person should provide sexual education for him. (Department of Health 1991b, Section 7.48)

In our interviews with local authority staff in component 1 no respondents were aware of any existing policy in this area but several reported that a policy was being formulated at the time of the interview. In practice it was seen as part of the responsibilities of residential carers or of educational support workers who visited residential homes to work with young people on health-related issues. In one authority a health educator for residential projects had recently been appointed. In another, a person had been appointed to carry out sexual health work with young people looked after (within the social services department), although she was employed by the local health commission. She reported that amongst the (very few) people in her position, the normal practice was for the appointment to be funded by a health authority within their HIV/AIDS budget rather than by a social services department. Furthermore, such appointments were usually made as short-term contracts which led to limited scope to engage in forward planning and continuity of input.

It was generally reported that young people being looked after in residential homes would have access to information about sex and contraception, although if their stay in the home were brief then they might well miss out on this aspect of education.

Work with individual young people was the domain of residential care workers in conjunction with case-holding social workers. In the *Looking After Children* materials, which most authorities were either using or planning to use, the Assessment and Action Records include areas to consider around sexual development, contraception and knowledge about relationships (Department of Health, 1991d). The use of these materials means that practice, at least, would be clearly defined. As one respondent pointed out, in this area of work policy frequently follows practice, rather than policy being clearly defined first.

Bremner and Hillin (1993) report that of the London boroughs and county councils in the London and south-east which they surveyed only one authority had trained residential staff in communicating with young people about sex. In our sample some provision was made for workers in residential homes to receive training in sex education and sexual health and some respondents referred to using material in the Guidance accompanying the Children Act (Department of Health, 1991b). Training did not take place within a policy framework but was typically carried out on an ad hoc basis and subject to the discretion of the individual home where levels of staffing were likely to dictate whether or not a worker could attend a course. Furthermore, training has in the past been somewhat urgently focused on sexual health, HIV and AIDS and this has tended to overshadow work on the avoidance of pregnancy.

Respondents in some authorities reported that they were in the process of formulating a general policy on health care for looked after young people of which sexual health was to be a part. The policy would also address training for residential carers. Consequently some progress on these issues might already have been made and in the interim a policy and practice framework for those working with children and young people in public care has already been published (Patel-Kanwal and Frances Lenderyou, 1998).

Where policy issues were being addressed these covered health and sex education. Sex education appears to be commonly subsumed under the heading of health issues and thus to be focused on sexual health and contraception. Furthermore, as we have already noted, relevant workers seemed to be employees of health authorities rather than social services departments. The report of a survey carried out by First Key in one local authority stated that young people's reporting of a lack of sex education and information about contraception should be a cause for concern and in fact might partly account for the high rate of parenthood amongst the sample. These comments appeared under the section relating to health, alongside comments on a sensible diet. While the point about lack of sex education is valid, its consideration might be better addressed under the umbrella term of relationships. Young people may be well aware of the need for protection against disease and pregnancy but may be unable to negotiate this with their partner. This theme will be further explored in the context of young people's responses.

The policies being formulated were targeted predominantly at residential homes. The position for foster carers remained largely unclear. Ideally foster carers should provide sex education as part of the work they are prepared to do with young people; in this sense the question as to whether they are providing it as parents or as professionals does not arise. They should have knowledge about sex education and relationships and be able to communicate this to those in their care. Most local authorities use the *Choosing to Foster* training material of which these issues are a part (National Foster Care Association, 1994). One respondent working in this area pointed out that pre-approval training means that 'a lot of subjects are touched on rather than covered in enormous depth'. Extra training would be provided for those looking after teenagers. Ongoing training is also available for foster carers on these and other topics, although such training is optional and, reportedly, take up is poor especially by those deemed to need it most. In one authority foster carers are routinely invited to join training courses run for social workers and residential care workers, a situation that, according to the respondent, would have been unheard of five or six years ago.

In one authority a training programme specifically for foster carers was piloted during 1995 following the appointment of a sexual health project worker with foster carers, a collaboration between the local council and health commission. In this authority the majority of children and young people being looked after are placed with foster carers. A system of accreditation for foster carers was being introduced and attendance at the five-day training programme on sexual health was to be compulsory.

The position of both residential and foster carers as regards the delivery of sex education to young people accommodated is not clear. Under the terms of the Children Act responsibility remains with parents unless there is a care order in effect. Carers who give contraceptive advice might feel they are stepping outside their boundaries. This underlines the importance of placement agreement meetings being held at which all parties involved in the welfare of the child or young person should be present. At these meetings the wishes of parents in respect of potentially delicate areas such as this can be ascertained, not only removing anxieties from the carers about imparting information on sex and contraception but also ensuring that young people do receive it. It was reported that in practice such meetings do not always take place. Bremner and Hillin (1993) pointed out that workers do have a responsibility to give advice, information and support to young people for this aspect of their lives but equally have the right to clear guidelines, policy and management support as well as the right to know what is expected of them.

It is not uncommon for social workers to find themselves inadvertently in a dilemma of the type described below.

'And someone else who did go on the pill when she was in care, she didn't want her mum to know and that put me in a really vulnerable position. We did seek legal advice, well they said it was actually the doctor who prescribes ... I mean I'd taken her ... – I think it was a pregnancy test I'd taken her to the GP for – and the next minute, he starts dishing out this pill, and there was absolutely no talk about safe sex; it was just, "Take this, it'll make you better. You won't get pregnant" sort of thing. And that was where it was left. And I had to be in the room while he was dishing out this prescription which really did put me in an awkward situation. And in the end the young woman told her mum.'

Sex education: experiences of young people

Sex education in schools

A large number of the young mothers and mothers-to-be who were interviewed in component 1 had not been regular school attenders and had finished their education completely by the age of 14. Thus many had at best only a hazy recollection of any sex education they had received in school and several stated that they had not received any. Others recalled that there may have been some but that they had not absorbed any of it since they had been in a permanent state of inattention at school. Those who could recall lessons on this topic were uniformly unimpressed by what they had received, summed up by one young woman's comment that 'school sex education is crap'. Their dissatisfaction covered timing, content, style and delivery. This account by an 18-year-old mother encapsulates all the aspects identified by other respondents.

> 'I think they give you it at the wrong age. Well they don't give you it at the wrong age but they do because they tell you things and it just makes you more, sort of ... I mean they start off with frogs, how frogs reproduce and things like that which at that age – 12, 13 – you find hilarious, you don't take it serious and they don't go into it. I remember the teacher telling us to write down all the sexual words we knew, then he went through them. He was embarrassed, because obviously kids would put everything down. And he didn't want to tell us about it, because it was real sort of explicit but ... I think that's what they do – they teach you about frogs having babies ... but not the sex as it is today. Not that type, what I think needs to be said, it's totally different from what you're taught.'

Pregnancy was routinely covered but not necessarily in a way that had meaning for the age group:

> 'They tell you how to get pregnant. But to 12, 13-year-old kids that don't mean nothing ... They just say – "Girls, when they start having their periods ..." But they do it in such a boring way.' (*18-year-old*)

Contraception was even less likely to be addressed and where it did feature in the syllabus the teaching was considered to be largely ineffective in preventing unprotected sexual activity:

'They showed you contraception and stuff like that. They have like a box, show you all these different contraceptions and that. "Well, the best way to have a baby is just to say no, that's the best contraception", but you just go out and do it anyway.' (laughs) (*19-year-old*)

One young woman summed up her school sex education as 'how to put a condom on a banana!'. She was clearly not impressed but she was, in fact, more fortunate than many whose education had consisted of a description of the reproductive system. Nevertheless, putting a condom on a banana teaches only a part of what young women need to know: it does not teach them how to negotiate contraceptive use with a possibly reluctant partner.

There was a general feeling that having someone other than a member of staff supply this aspect of education would be preferable. This would alleviate their own embarrassment over the topic and would allow them to ask questions of someone whom they did not have to meet on a regular basis and in a different context.

'Sex education really needs to be changed. They don't want these boring straight-laced teachers ... I think if you've got somebody who's sat there and you know you can't embarrass them, you wouldn't do it. I think somebody who teaches sex education should be somebody who comes into the school, not somebody who's there ... Some of my friends were pregnant very young and I think if somebody had sat down with us like that, it would've prevented it.' (*18-year-old*)

Thomson and Scott (1992) in their survey of local education authorities' provision referred to lack of confidence on the part of the teacher as a major problem in delivering effective sex education. Although training in this field has been inadequate and Department for Education and Employment guidance stresses the need for training to be reviewed, nevertheless the limited funding in schools for in-service training has not been sufficient to meet all requirements.

It was a general view of the young mothers interviewed that by the time the school began to give information about sex most of them had acquired the basic knowledge for themselves. The main sources of this knowledge were friends, books and the media. Not all of this was reliable nor was it necessarily well understood. Nevertheless, there was a widespread belief, often shared by component 2 respondents, that school sex education had little to add to their existing knowledge base.

The information on sex education obtained from the young people in component 2 is not directly comparable to that obtained from the young mothers in component 1. Data from the latter were collected some 18 months before those from the former and, furthermore, the average age of the component 2 sample was younger than that of the component 1 sample. The two sets of respondents might, therefore, have received their sex education some four or five years apart and have been subject not only to variations according to the school but also according to current thinking and delivery of sex education.

However, we can make direct comparisons between the samples in component 2, that is, between the young people in the care of a local authority and those living with their families, to establish whether those living in public care fared any worse than those who were not. The questionnaire contained a substantial question on topics that might have been covered in school sex education to which respondents were asked to reply whether the information had been given too early, too late, at the right time or not at all. Some topics relating to family life and child care are discussed more fully in the relevant chapters.

Looking first at the proportions answering 'not given any information on this topic' we see that in general the looked after sample does fare worse than the school sample, and there are particular areas where a notable difference is observed. In addition to family life and child care, these are: physical changes in adolescence, contraception, pregnancy, emergency contraception, pressure to have sex and sexual abuse. Moreover, the differences between the girls in the two samples are especially marked on some of these and are significant in respect of pregnancy and emergency contraception. Also noteworthy is the gap between the boys on pressure to have sex. While 13 per cent of the school sample boys said they had not been informed about this at school, the proportion of looked after boys in the same position was 23 per cent. Given that a large proportion of looked after boys considered that girls put pressure on boys to have sex (see Chapters 3 and 6), this would appear to be of significance for many.

In contrast, the looked after sample, and especially the girls, appeared to be notably better informed than the school sample about abortion and about accessing local health services.

For 12 of the 17 topics more than one third of the looked after sample said they had not received information at the right time: family life, child care, emergency contraception, animal reproduction, sexual feelings and emotions, pregnancy, sexually transmitted diseases, abortion, gay, lesbian and bisexual issues, using local health services, pressure to have sex, and sexual abuse and sexual violence. Nevertheless this is a better result than that for the school sample where more than one third claimed not have received information at the right time on all 17 topics.

Sex education in care

According to the young mothers and mothers-to-be in component 1, sex and contraception were not addressed routinely in residential care in a group setting. Where discussion did take place the focus was more likely to be contraception than sex and to be on a personal rather than group basis. Some young people reported that they could have asked carers if they wanted and some carers did use opportunities to talk individually with young people, though this was dependent on catching the young person 'in a good (that is, receptive) mood.' Not all young people wanted information or advice from carers and some were suspicious of their help. As one young mother pointed out, a great deal hinged on the nature of the relationship between staff and resident: if it was open and comfortable then a dialogue on this topic was much more likely to take place. Another indicated that her former fellow residents had been at pains to avoid talking to staff about these matters except in special circumstances:

> 'A lot of them used to, but only in front of everyone to try and get the staff embarrassed. Not out of any real need for information, just to wind the staff up.' (*17-year-old*)

Two respondents showed empathy for the position of carers and illustrated why they may have wished to avoid approaching the topic with a group of residents:

> 'I don't know if it's because they couldn't be bothered because they knew them lot wouldn't have gone anyway. I couldn't imagine our ones sitting down talking about contraception and sex. They'd probably've just sat there going, "Yeah, I did that last night with this girl down the road." It wouldn't have surprised me if they (staff) probably thought "No. I'll give that a miss!".' (*19-year-old*)

> 'I think it's actually a bit difficult for staff to say things at the right time. It all depends on the individual really, I think, because I know at that age if you're talking about things like that to a teenager, unless you know them really well and they can trust in you, then I think it's a dodgy situation because there's a lot of tearaways in care that won't listen to anything they've got to say.' (*18-year-old*)

Her proposed solution was to have information stored in a cupboard so that residents could either read it privately or could ask to go through it with a member of staff. This was reiterated by another respondent who had lived a great deal of her life in residential care and was aware of the need for information.

Sex education from parents

It has sometimes been assumed that those who are looked after by a local authority are at a particular disadvantage in learning about sex and contraception compared with young people living at home with parents who would impart this information. This is not necessarily the case. Parents often consider that their own sex education has been inadequate and that they would like some guidance on how to deliver this to their own children. Many feel uncomfortable talking to their children about sex, not only because they feel that their own knowledge may be incomplete but also because of the changing nature of the parent–child relationship during adolescence (Holland, Mauthner and Sharpe, 1996).

Of the young women in component 1 who had been living with their mother during their early teens, the majority reported that they had been given no information about sex, even if they had been told about contraception.

> 'I mean, my mum talked to me about contraception, she never talked to me about sex. She only went round it.' (*18-year-old*)

> 'I can always remember when I was about 11 I went to my mum's friend's house and she had this book about sex, *The Joy of Sex* or something. And I remember I stole it. And my friend told my mum so I got a smack. I don't think she should've smacked me ... I always wanted to ask my mum. I was always curious about it.' (*16-year-old*)

Yet this young woman's mother had, apparently, had no difficulty in talking about or taking a liberal stance on contraception, or indeed, on sexual activity amongst young people in general.

Sometimes the lack of information had alarming or distressing consequences. One 16-year-old who had spent many years with the same foster carers was not allowed by her carers to attend school sex education lessons, nor was she given any information at home.

> 'Parents had to sign a form saying you could watch videos and stuff. And my foster parents wouldn't sign ... No, they didn't tell me nothing. I just learnt it all through experience ... I didn't even know what a period was till it were there ... I just went in the bath and then I went to the shop and just bought what I had to buy.'

She ran away from her carers and became pregnant at the age of 15. By the time she was 16 she was living alone with her baby in a council flat.

Another 16-year-old, also pregnant at 15, described the panic associated with a lack of information:

> 'My mother always refused to answer any questions we had about sex so I learned it all from magazines and then went to the library to get some books so I could learn a bit more. Now she's refusing to give my youngest sister any information. She recently started her periods and thought she was going to bleed to death.'

In component 2 an identical question to the one on sex education in school covered information from parents and/or carers. The purpose of this question was not to establish whether it was parents or carers who gave information about sex and relationships to looked after young people but rather to examine how they compared with their non-looked after peers in terms of receiving information in their 'home' setting.

With the exception of family life and child care (where, as we discuss elsewhere, the looked after sample was at a disadvantage), the only major difference in terms of not being given any information was that the girls in public care were far less likely than the girls in the school sample to have been told about body changes in puberty, supporting the comments of the young mothers in component 1. But in terms of the time at which they were given information there were two important areas of significant difference between the girls: more in the looked after sample than the school sample thought that they had been told *too late* about sexual feelings and emotions and about pressure to have sex.

For looked after boys in terms of not having been given any information, the only areas of particular disadvantage were regarding sexual feelings and emotions and accessing local health services; the difference between them and the school sample boys falls just short of significance. But in respect of the timing of the delivery of information, the boys in public care were significantly more likely than the school sample boys to say that they had been told *too early* by parents or carers both about sexual relationships and about sexual feelings and emotions.

In interviews with the school sample several young people said that they learned all they needed to know about sex from parents while others relied on them for information about what they described as the 'emotional and mental' side of sex which, they claimed, was not taught at school. However, there was such variation in the responses about what information was given by parents that no conclusion can be drawn about the function of parents as educators in this respect.

Effectiveness of sex education

From the replies to the questions on school sex education and information from parents in component 2, it would seem that there were still relatively high proportions of young people with an average age of 15, whether looked after or not, whose parents or carers had not talked to them about: contraception, pregnancy, emergency contraception, HIV and AIDS, sexually transmitted diseases, gay, lesbian and bisexual issues, accessing local health services, pressure to have sex and sexual abuse.

Further analysis was carried out to establish whether those who had not been given information at school on these topics had also not been told about them by parents or carers, comparing respondents from the two samples. For four topics the proportion in the school sample who had not having been given information either at school or from parents slightly exceeded that of the looked after sample: gay, lesbian and bisexual relationships, accessing local health services, abortion, and relationships with the opposite sex. For all the other topics the looked after sample respondents outnumbered the school sample respondents in respect of not having been given information. Within the looked after sample there was generally little difference between the genders.

Where information had been given, for most variables it was given less often 'at the right time' at home or in care than it was in school, suggesting that school sex education is capable of being appropriately timed. Where information was not given at the right time it was more likely to have been given too late rather than too early, with the notable exceptions of sexual intercourse and pregnancy which a proportion of both samples felt they had been told about at home or in care too early.

In the component 2 samples there was a high level of agreement that knowing the facts about sex and contraception makes young people more careful, although this was lowest among the looked after girls and highest among school sample boys (Table A.1, Appendix B). But some ambivalence in attitude was observed in the looked after sample as a whole, where an equal proportion (73 per cent) also thought that such knowledge would make them more likely to experiment. In the school sample only 61 per cent thought experimenting would result from increased knowledge but many more boys (71 per cent), who had earlier stated that knowledge makes young people more careful, than girls (50 per cent) thought this was the case. An identical proportion (71 per cent) of girls in the looked after sample agreed that knowledge about sex and contraception leads to experimentation though this was not the view of the young mothers in component 1. This reflects the public debate about whether sex education is responsible for delaying or promoting sexual activity.

The young mothers in the component 1 sample considered that too little sex education is more harmful than too much and that increased knowledge would not lead to increased activity. Most considered that having too little information was far more problematical than having too much. Being fed snippets of information and relying on friends for what were often incorrect facts could lead to far greater dangers than being well informed.

> 'I think if you don't know – they give you a little bit and then you just want to find out more, it leads you the wrong way. Whereas if you knew it all, you'd think, "Oh well...".' (*16-year-old*)

Being told the stark facts not only about sex but about the outcome of unprotected sex might have led some young women down a different path:

> 'If it had been done at all properly in school, I reckon, after seeing it and knowing all the details, it might have put me off. I might have been more stricter on it.' (*16-year-old, pregnant at 14*)

> 'I would certainly have had second thoughts if someone had told me that it's not going to turn out how you see it. I think I would have definitely thought twice.' (*19-year-old, first pregnant at 13*)

But this may be only part of the picture. The only young woman in the sample to have received what she considered to be effective sex education at school, and who in addition had received a great deal of information from her mother, was still unintentionally pregnant at the age of 16. Another part of the picture may be the less easy task of persuading young people that they are not invincible. Knowledge of the facts may simply not be enough:

> 'It doesn't matter what you know. People know about contraception and that ... I don't think people take it as serious as they should be taking it.' (*17-year-old, pregnant at 16*)

> 'People could've spent their lives telling me to be careful because one day... and I would've thought "I don't think so. Not now.".' (*Pregnant 17-year-old*)

Among the young people in component 2 there was a general belief in both samples that sex education was adequate and that lack of knowledge about sex was not a reason for teenage pregnancy.

> 'I mean, it's taught in schools from, what, the age of 10. And it's taught every year until you reach year 9. So if they haven't got it through to them, then they never will.' (*Female*)

It was also backed up by information from other sources:

> '... everyone is educated.'
> 'Everyone knows, even if your mum doesn't sit you down and tell you and talk about sex with you, you always pick it up off the streets ...'
> 'I don't think you pick it up from TV very much. I think even if your Mum and Dad and teachers are open about it, I think you know all about it before they talk to you, because of your friends.'
>
> (*Mixed school group*)

Apart from school and home, other sources of information were friends, magazines and siblings. One young woman reported that she always asked her older brother for information because she would feel too embarrassed to discuss the topic with her parents. She thought her parents were relieved that her brother would act as her source of information. Girls in particular found magazines to be a good source of information. In a school discussion group two young women discussed the value of teenage magazines

> 'Magazines, I think they're very good. I don't think they overrate sex or anything, they're very informative and helpful. The problem pages, I really enjoy reading.'
> 'I don't think you learn as much from TV.'

However, one young man in another school discussion group with two young women opined that 'Some girls might read magazines that are too old for them' to which one of the girls responded, 'Yeah, but we do and it doesn't influence us!'. Nevertheless in response to the earlier question about pressure to form relationships, the school sample respondents had been much more likely than those from public care to think that magazines were a source of pressure on girls to have a boyfriend.

Another major source of information for many in the school sample was television 'confessional' programmes which, and particularly the more extreme American versions, occupied something of a cult status among pupils. They were, apparently, watched daily and their content discussed in detail the following day at school. This, they stated, was their main, and preferred, way of learning about relationships.

> 'It's hard to learn a lot about relationships from magazines.'
> 'We find out about that stuff from TV shows like XYZ ... It's always got relationships and breaking up and all that. (To interviewer) You should watch it, Miss.'
> **Would you use it for discussion in a lesson?** (*Researcher*)
> 'Oh no. He (teacher) would probably be annoyed that we were talking about it.'
> **What makes this a good way of learning about relationships?** (*Researcher*)
> 'Because people have experienced it.'
> 'And they explain how they feel and how they're coping and it's better than just reading about it in a magazine. You can actually feel how they feel.'
> 'You can scream and shout and that (as the studio audience does).'
> 'It's probably more extreme because it's American. But there's, like, ABC. That's an English talk show but it's not as good.'
> 'It deals with things like how a man had an affair and his wife took him back.'
> 'It's simple, like. XYZ is more complicated.'
> 'A man who's got two wives or a man who loves another man, or transvestites.'
> 'And there's fighting.'
>
> (*Mixed school group*)

The young people in this group further considered that this would be their ideal way of learning about everything to with sex and relationships, and an effective way of dealing with the issue of teenage pregnancy:

> 'It might be a show about contraception and they'd have someone who had a kid when she was 15 and it would be about how they feel and what they would have gone through and how hard it was.'
> **And would that be a deterrent?** (*Researcher*)
> 'Not all the time.'

'Depends how good the show was. If the show was good you're never going to forget it.'
'It's better than the teacher telling you, "No, don't do it".'
'You're bound to do the opposite of what the teacher says.'

In fact what they were advocating was peer education which is already carried out in schools by young mothers in some areas of the country. They were united in believing that this would be a more effective method than the teacher simply passing on information, and that equally effective would be someone aged 16 to 19 who had a child coming into the school to talk to them about pregnancy.

'Because they've experienced it.'
'Because they know what the modern day's like, and that's how we work.'
'Because teachers haven't, like, experienced having kids at a young age but that person would have.'
They might have ... (*Researcher*)
'No. They're too sensible!'
'And the teachers you already know, and the more you get to know them you don't want to talk about things like that.'
'It does depend on the teacher. You have to trust the teacher. But if you don't know the teacher that well you wouldn't want to talk to them.'
'And if it's a female teaching the boys it might be more difficult but if it's a male teaching the girls it's all right.'

A residential care worker in the component 1 sample reported that young mothers often return to the independent living unit where she works and 'preach' to current residents, telling them 'Don't be stupid, go out, get a job and do this and do that' to little effect. She added, 'And I look at them and they say, "We know. Why did we do this?". But I don't say anything.'

Contraception

Having explored the extent to which young people are given reliable information about sex and relationships we now examine the attitudes and access to contraception of looked after young people and their experiences of different methods.

Attitudes to contraception

Most of the young mothers and mothers-to-be in component 1 considered that young people do not worry about contraception, or not until it is too late. This is, to some extent, confirmed in the findings from component 2, where only about one third of the young people reported that they 'always' worried about themselves or their girlfriend becoming pregnant. A lower proportion of respondents in the looked after sample (30 per cent) than in the school sample (38 per cent) said that they were always worried, with boys least likely to do so (23 per cent). Likewise the proportion of looked after girls (36 per cent) who always worried was considerably lower than that of their counterparts in the school sample (42 per cent). Just over half of all respondents said that they 'sometimes' worried about the possibility of pregnancy, with girls in the looked after sample most likely to report this and looked after boys least likely.

Consequently the looked after boys was the group most likely to state that they did 'not usually' worry about pregnancy. As many as 30 per cent of them claimed this was their position, compared with only 4 per cent of the looked after girls, an identical proportion to that of the school sample girls. The comparable proportion of school sample boys is 15 per cent, indicating that there is a disparity between the genders in the extent of their concern.

On the basis of this evidence it would seem that boys in public care, even more than those who are not in care, are frequently ignoring the possible consequences of their actions. Looked after girls appeared to be more concerned than boys but were not as consistently worried as their peers who are not looked after.

Teenagers are more likely than any other age group to engage in short-term sexual relationships and those aged 17 and under are far less likely than women in the older age groups to take any precautions (Mellanby, Phelps and Tripp, 1993; Wellings and others, 1994; Office of Population Censuses and Surveys, 1995a). The precise proportions not using any form of contraception vary according to the study, from 50 per cent of women under 16 (Wellings and others, 1994) to around 70 per cent of 16- and 17-year-olds (Office of Population Censuses and Surveys, 1995).

The young women in component 1 of this study proved to be no exception to the statistics, which imply that they frequently run the risk of becoming pregnant. Many of them reported using no method of contraception though only one had done so in the mistaken belief that she would not become pregnant on the first occasion of intercourse. However, since this view was related by her mother rather than the young woman herself, and since she had subsequently had two more children before reaching the age of 20, its veracity is by no means certain. No others claimed to have acted out of ignorance.

Experience of contraception

In component 1 the sample of young mothers appeared to be divided between those who used no method of contraception and those who used a method that failed.

No method of contraception

Firstly, there was a small number of young women who were overtaken by events and had not really paused to ponder the implications of their acts. Alcohol, traditionally associated with a decreased likelihood of contraceptive use (Leigh, 1990), may have played a part. The situation was most likely to have arisen when an existing friendship or casual encounter turned into sexual activity.

> 'It was just the situation at the time – we were just friends – and then I was pregnant. I would've used contraception under different circumstances.' (*18-year-old, pregnant at 17*)

Secondly, there was a larger number who did not use any form of protection as a result of their belief that they were unassailable.

> 'At 16 I really thought I was invincible. I thought "Nothing is going to happen to me, I can fight it off".' (*17-year-old, pregnant at 16*)

> 'Nobody could tell me anything. I knew everything.' (*15-year-old, pregnant at 14*)

This conviction was strengthened by the fact that previous episodes of unprotected sex had not resulted in a pregnancy. When asked if they had been concerned about becoming pregnant these young women typically replied along the following lines:

> 'I thought there was probably something wrong with one of us. I never expected it to happen ... I'd got away with it for so long it just wasn't even on my mind ... If nothing happens you don't expect it ever to happen.' (*17-year-old, pregnant*)

> 'You just don't think really, do you? You just ... don't think. "I've got away with it before," you think, "I'll get away with it now."' (*17-year-old, pregnant at 16*)

For a very small number of others, however, doing nothing was a positive choice. Even if they did not explicitly want to be pregnant they were certainly not averse to the idea and for them not using contraception was a form of casting fate to the winds. As one 17-year-old with a considerable amount of self-awareness stated, 'I don't think I minded being pregnant, otherwise I would have taken the necessary precautions in the first place.'

None of the young women stated that they had failed to protect themselves out of fear of being labelled promiscuous. Their views on pressures to have boyfriends and sexual relationships set out previously indicate that they largely inhabited a world in which sexual activity was the norm and there was, therefore, no danger of being criticised for being either experienced or prepared. Only 14 per cent of the girls in component 2 agreed with the statement that 'women who carry condoms sleep around'.

Condoms

For those who chose to use some form of protection the condom appeared to be the most favoured method. Young people use condoms more frequently than those in any other age group (Brook Advisory Centres, 1995; Office of Population Censuses and Surveys, 1995; Health Education Authority, 1996). In this sample its popularity may be due to its general availability which does not require a young person to consult with social workers or carers before using it. In addition, some residential care staff, concerned to protect young people from disease and pregnancy, do supply young people with condoms.

After-care centres often keep supplies of condoms in obvious places and encourage young people to help themselves. One after-care worker reported that:

> 'We have a never-ending supply of condoms in our office, and if we know our young people are sexually active then I usually find I'm popping them in their pockets if I know they're not picking them up.'

Condom use declines with age but it also declines with familiarity. As relationships develop other methods are more likely to be chosen. It was not seen as a long-standing contraceptive arrangement for the young women in this sample and was likely to be replaced by another method once a relationship became established. Several young women reported that they were about to turn to the contraceptive pill or the injection (Depo-Provera) when they discovered they were pregnant. They may also have decided simply to discontinue use without adopting another method, especially if their initial concerns had centred around protection from disease rather than avoidance of pregnancy.

Given an average failure of two in every 100, condoms had a relatively high failure rate amongst the users in this group of young people. However, information supplied by the Family Planning Association suggests that splitting and bursting of condoms is more common than is acknowledged on the basis of the number of resulting pregnancies, and in a study of patients requesting a termination of pregnancy (Bromham and Cartmill, 1993) it was suggested that over the last 20 years the number of unplanned pregnancies connected to condom use has increased.

One possible explanation is incorrect use, while another may be the quality of condoms supplied in children's homes which was reported to be not very good. One young woman reported that it would have been pointless to use the condoms they were given because they always burst. Yet another explanation is that young women who attributed their pregnancy to condom failure may in fact have been using no method at all. If they had already made it clear in the interview that they were fully aware of the facts about conception and contraception, as they invariably did, then it might have been less embarrassing to attribute their mistake to circumstances outside their control. Not all young women were as confident as the 17-year-old who, when asked whether she had been using any form of contraceptive replied, 'No, I wasn't, and I'm not ashamed to say that either'.

Oral contraceptives

The other method of contraception frequently used by the young women in the sample was the pill. This is the most popular method amongst single women and the most frequently used by those aged 16–24 years, two thirds of whom reported use in the previous year (Office of Population Censuses and Surveys, 1995). For the young women in our study oral contraception seemed to be a favoured method where they had sought or been offered advice from a social worker, residential worker or staff at a clinic. However, memory and side-effects inhibited its use. Several young women reported forgetting to take it. Disruption and disorganisation were features of many young women's lives and worked against them doing anything on a regular and routine basis. If they were 'scatterbrained', as one young person described herself, then their living circumstances compounded the problem.

'I were either forgetting to take the pill or taking it at different times.' (*17-year-old, pregnant at 16*)

'I was on pill, but then I came off it because I kept forgetting to take it.' (*18-year-old, pregnant at 17*)

'It was all this moving around, moving doctors, I couldn't get it and things, I just forgot about it.' (*17-year-old, pregnant at 16*)

Another young woman, aware of the need to take the pill at a specific time each day with little leeway, attributed her forgetfulness to the lack of routine in her life. She had always taken the pill at lunchtime at school but once her life became disrupted and she did not attend school then the routine was lost. Having resumed the use of the pill after the birth of her child she commented that having her own accommodation ('at least I always wake up in the same place now') meant that she could leave the contraceptives in an obvious place and thus never forgot them.

Side-effects associated with oral contraceptives discouraged others from continuing to take them:

'I was on the pill, but I just couldn't take to it. I was being sick, they tried all different ones because I was being sick.' (*16-year-old, pregnant at 14*)

One had had additional difficulty in obtaining medical advice and attention when she had experienced adverse side-effects and this had led to her discontinuing use and becoming pregnant:

'I got all the side-effects from it so I went to the doctors to try and get it changed. But he didn't want to know, because I didn't get it from him. So I just gave it up altogether.' (*17-year-old, pregnant*)

In one case a young woman discovered too late that the pill was not effective for her:

'I found out afterwards that my mum couldn't take the pill neither, it didn't work for her. It was a bit late afterwards. So I thought I was being really careful, but I wasn't, obviously.' (*18-year-old, pregnant at 17*)

Forgetfulness and problems associated with side-effects of the pill may lead to pregnancy, but so may lack of information on the extent to which gastrointestinal upsets and the use of antibiotics can impair efficacy. An after-care worker pointed out:

'They don't realise that if they have a tummy bug and they're taking the pill they can get pregnant. It can be a genuine accident.'

In a study carried out amongst women with an unplanned pregnancy about half of those using an oral contraceptive said that they had received no instructions about what to do if they had medical problems or if they missed taking a pill (Duncan and others, 1990) and one fifth of them were aware of the need to take further precautions but had not done so. Another study pointed to the high proportion of women taking the pill who did not know which factors led to diminished efficacy (Brook and Smith, 1991). Brook Advisory Services do provide a leaflet but inevitably this cannot address individual levels of literacy, familiarity with the language and ability to absorb written information.

Lack of information combined with lack of understanding could account for a considerable number of these, and similar, unintended pregnancies amongst young women (Phoenix, 1991). According to Fleissig's study the incidence of unintended pregnancies amongst pill users increased during the 1980s. This may have been partly due to more recently developed forms of the pill, some of which are only just strong enough to prevent pregnancy and require careful usage and, therefore, careful explanation (Fleissig, 1991). One young woman in our sample reported becoming pregnant when, having experienced adverse reactions to a previous contraceptive, she had been given one 'that wasn't strong enough or something.'

A study amongst 744 women aged between 16 and 49 carried out by the Contraceptive Education Service in 1996, and reported in *The Guardian* newspaper on 14 February 1996, found that 40 per cent of women considered that they were not given as much information as they would like about possible side-effects and nearly a quarter specifically wanted more information about thrombosis. The occasional publication of data highlighting symptoms such as the increased risk of thrombosis associated with some types of oral contraception serves to increase women's awareness of potential, as well as actual, problems. These so-called 'pill scares' can lead to women ceasing to take the pill without using another form of protection according to a report from the British Pregnancy Advisory Service quoted in *The Guardian* on 15 April 1996. When the media choose to stress the adverse effects without presenting the benefits, women may react by panicking and by considering that they have been kept in the dark about the potential harm to themselves. It also prompts fears of an increase in the rate of teenage pregnancy. Young people living alone in the community with no one to consult may be particularly at risk of reacting in this way and leaving themselves unprotected. One possible reason for the latest increase in teenage conceptions which appears in the statistics for 1996 (Office for National Statistics, 1998b) is a 'pill scare' towards the end of the previous year.

Other methods

The injection and implant appear to be becoming favoured methods. They have advantages over many alternatives in that they do not rely on memory or correct usage on each occasion of intercourse. They do, however, produce side-effects of even greater magnitude and higher incidence than those associated with the oral contraceptive (Stacey, 1990). One young woman described how the contraceptive injection had made her ill tempered so she had returned to using the pill which caused her to put on weight, adding 'I'd rather be fat than grumpy.' Others experienced reactions far in excess of grumpiness:

> 'I did have the injection which was given to me and nothing suited me. I just kept on haemorrhaging and haemorrhaging.' (*16-year-old, pregnant at 14*)

> 'After having him I had the injection as a contraception and never stopped bleeding from it. I came off it and I'm still bleeding now. I'm on a course of tablets, have to go and see a gynaecologist and see what damage is done. I just have to wait and find out.' (*18-year-old, pregnant at 15*)

> 'I've had the implant put in my arm, I can't have any more until he's five ... Yeah, I was a bit ill with them at first. I've been to doctors loads of times, got rushed to hospital once. I had inflamed ovaries and kidneys from side-effects of these implants. But I had tablets after I came out of hospital so I've been all right. They've been in a year now. It's settled down now ... It was (bad) at the time. It didn't last for long, it was like a day and a half I was like that. But other than that, not really. Put a bit of weight on.' (*19-year-old, pregnant at 17*)

As related by the young women concerned, these side-effects appeared to be played down, perhaps because they considered this a fair price to pay for avoiding another pregnancy or perhaps because they were not used to taking decisions about themselves and consequently had a greater acceptance of suffering than would be found in the wider population.

Only one young women had received advice against using this method which she was probably more willing than many to heed since she had previously, under considerable pressure, had a termination.

'I was going to go for the injection, the one I was going to have was every three months. But then I was going to the family planning clinic about that, where my mum worked, the doctor turned round and said that it's better not to have an injection because of being so young, sometimes it can stop you having kids and can affect you inside. I don't know what it does. It can affect you inside, it can really muddle you up sometimes. She says "You can go for it if you want but I'm just warning you now. I'm just going to tell you the downside of it".' (*16-year-old, pregnant at 14*)

Nevertheless, these methods appeared to be constantly recommended, sometimes with considerable urgency, to young women in this sample who had had at least one child. One 15-year-old reported that while she was in hospital 'they rushed me in two days after I'd had him and they said, "Have you thought about contraception?" I said, "No, not yet", and they gave me an injection'. One foster carer looking after a 15-year-old with a baby reported, with some sense of relief, that the young mother was already using this form of contraception when she came to live with them but that she did prompt her to go for the repeat injections because she would otherwise forget. She did not necessarily view this as a part of her responsibility towards N but admitted that she was 'scared of the consequences' and added, 'Whether she's active or whether she isn't, I'm not taking that risk!'.

Those who used this method, and some who did not, thought that it was effective because 'taking the pill you can quite easily forget that but if you are going to inject it then you don't have to worry if you haven't took the pill and you might be pregnant' (*19-year-old*). One after-care worker said that they did suggest it to young women 'if they were unsure about taking the pill'.

Emergency contraception

Emergency contraception (the morning-after pill) was used only by one young woman who, having tried various other methods without success, used this on a regular, though reportedly not frequent, basis. For the other young women, using emergency contraception was not really an issue for the reasons discussed above: the belief that they would not or could not become pregnant either because they were invincible or because previous accidents with or non-use of contraception had not led to pregnancy. The shock to these young women of discovering that they were pregnant, described later, bears out their belief that they could engage in unprotected sexual intercourse without any cause for anxiety. Emergency contraception was not something they would have turned to, simply because they had not considered that they would conceive. In addition, as we noted earlier, girls in public care appeared to be much less well informed about emergency contraception than those in the school sample.

Accessing contraceptive services

The issue of contraception is addressed in the health section of the assessment and action records which form part of the *Looking After Children* documents for those aged ten years and over (Department of Health, 1995b). This gives young people the option to decline or to request further input and allows them to specify from whom they would like further help. However, it is not clear that young people use this opportunity nor would they necessarily wish to as they typically complete the forms with their social workers. In addition, while clearly there are opportunities to discuss contraception outside of the planning scenario, we have already noted that, without practice guidelines and training, social workers and carers may feel uneasy about offering advice on contraception, let alone contraception itself.

For the young women in component 1, the main sources of contraception were reported to be Brook Advisory Centres and family planning clinics, the latter providing a domiciliary service at one of the mother-and-baby units in the study. General practitioners were infrequently consulted. But many of the young women sought contraceptive advice when they were, or believed they might be, already pregnant.

'So, I decided not to (have the injection) and by then I'd found out I was pregnant. So it was too late.' *(16-year-old, pregnant for the second time at 15)*

'I'd actually gone down to the family clinic to see about the pill and they gave me some ... "Wait for your first period to come along, start taking them" – and that period never came.' *(18-year-old, pregnant at 15)*

This is not an uncommon event among young women generally: a pregnancy scare is often needed to prompt young people to go for contraceptive advice (Meyrick and Harris, 1995).

A problem for carers and social workers lies in getting right the timing of ensuring that young people are not at risk of unwanted pregnancy without incurring allegations of encouraging sexual activity. In some cases in our study social workers reported that they were about to arrange a visit to the family planning clinic for their young clients when they had already discovered they were pregnant.

'She (social worker) did give me a lecture about having some sort of contraception. It was obvious I was having sex when I went for the pregnancy test. She took me to get the pill though I knew I was pregnant.' (*15-year-old, pregnant at 14*)

This goes some way towards contradicting the fairly widespread belief among some members of the public and press that all social workers and residential carers offer contraceptive advice or supply contraception indiscriminately to young people so that they might engage in under-age sexual activity. Some, in fact, not only do not take their clients for contraception but, according to the young women, do not even discuss sex and contraception with them. However, in some cases this may be due to the fact that the young person herself prevents any discussion taking place. One social worker for a 15-year-old who was pregnant at the age of 14 reported that 'When her mum told me that she thought T was sexually active I did have a word with her, but she just laughed.' Others do address the issue:

'It's not that contraception's not on the agenda ... I just ram it down their throat!'

'We still talk about it and have a laugh and a joke about it.'

'I don't know if it was ever covered formally, it could well have been. It was covered in visits. Myself and P (key worker in residential home), we talked about contraception with G ... But nothing on a formal basis, it was more informal of talking through issues of contraception with G on routine visits. We did address it, obviously not good enough, but we did!'

Some social workers appeared to take young women to family planning clinics only when they were certain that they had become sexually active, though this carried the risk of it being too late.

'When N was coming out of the secure unit, because she's on a care order I took her to a well woman clinic, to seek advice. But she was already pregnant at that point.' (*Social worker for 15-year-old, pregnant at 14*)

'She was due to go to the Brook and we found out she was pregnant so it's just so ironic ...' (*Social worker for 16-year-old, pregnant at 15*)

'I usually know what she's taking, though obviously I didn't when she got pregnant.' (*Social worker for 16-year-old, pregnant at 14*)

This social worker had recently accompanied the young mother to a Brook Advisory Centre. She reported that she went as a friend, not as a social worker: firstly, because if she went in her social worker capacity Brook would make a charge to the social services department and, secondly, she considered it preferable for the young woman because it gave her 'the right message about getting free advice and help for herself.'

In one case a young woman, who had already been pregnant while in a residential home, was refused permission to start taking an oral contraceptive:

> 'I know in the home I asked to go on the pill but they weren't going to do it. They wouldn't let you go on the pill, obviously because I wasn't old enough, so I suppose they didn't let you go on it.' (*19-year-old*)

Some young women deplored the fact that workers were aware that sexual activity was taking place between young people in residential care but did nothing to ensure that young people had any form of protection from either pregnancy or disease. These were comments from young women in two different local authorities:

> 'In a children's home ... they must know where there are teenagers in a place like that, they need some information or someone there to talk to ... All the kids in the home, when they knew I was pregnant, they didn't hide the fact that they were sleeping together and still they (carers) did nothing about contraception there.' (*19-year-old*)

> 'I was talking to one of the staff who works at X (residential boarding school) and he says it's a tricky situation because even though everybody's doing it they cannot issue condoms. Some of them are 15 and that, they've got to have permission to be on the pill and that.' (*17-year-old*)

Being able to obtain contraception without having to advertise the fact to parents or carers is an important aspect for all young people but possibly more important for those who feel that their lives have largely been taken over by others:

> 'If you wanted to go on the pill they would have to have known about it and you don't want them knowing about something like that, at that age (14), do you?' (*19-year-old*)

One 15-year-old, in a placement 'in the middle of nowhere', was aware that she could get the pill from a family planning clinic but could not get there without her carers knowing. Another reported that when she was about 13 or 14 she had gone to her local family planning clinic only to be told that she needed her mother's permission before she could be given the pill.

As we noted earlier, many young people had not been given information at school about accessing local services and even more reported that this was not a topic talked about with carers or parents. While more girls in the looked after sample than those in the school sample had been given information by parents or carers, the reverse was true of the looked after boys compared with the boys in the school sample. Nevertheless as many as 83 per cent of those in the looked after sample (compared with 74 per cent in the school sample) agreed with the statement 'It's easy for young people to get contraceptives'.

Lack of knowledge either about where to obtain contraception or the need to use it were not considered by young people to be the most likely causes of unintended pregnancies (see Chapter 6). But, as with the mothers in component 1, these young people generally believed that knowledge was not always transformed into practice. There are many reasons for this including carelessness, invincibility, and alcohol and drugs which impair judgement at critical stages.

In addition, discussing contraception with a new partner requires a degree of confidence which young people in general and those looked after in particular do not always possess. In the component 2 quantitative study, 39 per cent of the looked after sample and 36 per cent of the school sample agreed that they would be too embarrassed to talk about contraception with a new partner. Girls, especially those in the school sample, were less likely than boys to feel embarrassed: 35 per cent of looked after girls and 29 per cent of school sample girls said they would be but over 40 per cent of all boys, with little difference between the samples, indicated that embarrassment would prevent them discussing contraception with a new girlfriend.

Preventing unplanned pregnancy

Although some level of ignorance remained, it is unlikely that the unplanned pregnancies in this sample could be attributed to a lack of knowledge. This confirms the findings of other research which concluded that most young women who become pregnant do not do so in a state of ignorance either about contraception or about how conception occurs (Phoenix, 1991). One social worker offered an explanation:

'Yes, yes she did (have reasonable knowledge). She's not stupid. No, she wasn't vulnerable, she wasn't taken advantage of, she was aware of, probably, what she was doing ... She said it was an accident. I don't know what I think about that ... because her mum had always been very good on contraception, very open minded but obviously she didn't choose to heed people's advice, she was just absolutely enjoying the freedom of being accommodated, just going off and doing whatever. Maybe she didn't know the consequences. Especially kids who are accommodated, they are just overwhelmed by not having to answer to parents any more and: "What are the consequences if I abscond for a few nights? When I come back what could possibly happen?".'

Another problem may relate to the attitude of young women. A social worker commented that her client had starting obtaining oral contraceptives at the age of 12 but probably 'did not know what she was doing with them.' It was a part of the belief system of 'I'm sexually active, I'd better be grown up sort of thing'.

The young women in component 1 consistently stressed the need for better education, for more information and for more emphasis to be placed on the need to use contraception and to use it properly.

> 'They should definitely give people under 16, you know, just give them condoms whether they're authorised or not, because it's definitely going on.' (*17-year-old*)

> 'At the end of the day if two people are going to have sex unless you cut off their vital organs ... there is nothing you can do to stop them, and it's better for them to be protected, to know what they are doing, than just be clueless.' (*17-year-old*)

> 'Just make sure you think about contraception wisely and if you're on pills, don't miss them.' (*16-year-old*)

Or, as one young man in a component 2 discussion group succinctly remarked, 'If you're gonna do it, at least do it safe'.

Lack of or inadequate use of contraception may be a function of how sex education in general is handled in the UK. In most teaching programmes it appears to be addressed as a question of health. While there is undoubtedly a health issue to be considered, an equally pressing one may be relationships and this is recognised in that section of the Guidance to the Children Act 1989 which addresses sex education for young people in public care:

> Sexual education will need to cover practical issues such as contraception ... However it must also cover the emotional aspects of sexuality, such as the part that sexuality plays in a young person's sense of identity; the emotional implications of entering into a sexual relationship with another person; and the need to treat sexual partners with consideration and not as objects to be used. (*Department of Health, 1991b, Section 7.49*)

Summary points

Many of the mothers and mothers-to-be interviewed in component 1 had not received any sex education at school, but those who had were critical of its timing (too late), its content (not covering essential topics) and its style of delivery (accompanied by embarrassment). They had not been compensated by receiving sex education from carers, who typically limited their input in this area to answering individual questions about contraception. But those young people who had lived at home before entering the care system in adolescence had not usually fared better in respect of receiving information from parents.

In component 2 the differences that emerged between the samples in respect of information received from parents and/or carers on a range of topics related to sex and relationships were important ones. Girls in public care were not told about physical changes associated with adolescence to the same extent as those living with their families were. They also felt that they had been told *too late* about pressure to have sex and about sexual feelings. The boys, on the other hand, thought that either they had not been told at all about sexual feelings or had been told *too early* and they also felt that they had been given information about sexual relationships too soon.

From lessons at school the looked after group, and especially the girls, were not so well informed as the school group on certain issues including contraception, pregnancy, emergency contraception, pressure to have sex and sexual abuse, and the differences between the girls were significant in respect of emergency contraception and pregnancy. A further major area of difference lay in the proportion of boys who had not learnt about pressure to have sex, which was much smaller in the looked after sample than in the school sample. This is important when considered alongside the findings which indicate that many looked after boys thought such pressure was placed on boys and young men by females.

Boys in public care were least likely to worry about a possible pregnancy and most likely to be too embarrassed to discuss contraception with a new partner. Some may still believe that contraception is a woman's responsibility: as one young man remarked, 'I reckon more girls should carry fammidoms, pappadums, femidoms – same thing'. But at the same time more than one third of all the boys in component 2 thought that women who carry condoms sleep around.

There was variation in the attitude of carers and social workers towards contraception and sexually active young people: while some advocated its use, others effectively denied young people the means to obtain it. Social workers often addressed the issue of protection too late to benefit their young clients. However, identifying the most appropriate time is not an easy task if charges of advocating premature sexual activity are to be avoided.

There are no grounds for believing that, overall, looked after young people are ignorant about sex and contraception. The information from component 2 confirms both young people's awareness of the need to use contraception and their somewhat cavalier attitude towards doing so, and this was a view endorsed by the young women in component 1. Where young people appear to suffer is in the application of their knowledge. In this sense they are probably not significantly different from their peers in the wider community who become pregnant unintentionally (Burghes, 1995). But for this sample a contributory factor for some may be a lack of confidence and self-esteem which renders it difficult for them to claim what they want in a relationship. Even more difficult would be negotiating with a partner over the delicate matter of the use of a condom, the most favoured method of contraception for this age group. Moore and Rosenthal (1993) indicate that open communication about wishes and needs is not a feature of teenage communication during a sexual encounter. However, the information from component 2 suggests that this is a bigger issue for looked after boys than it is for looked after girls. Great progress has been made in persuading young people to obtain condoms but perhaps they, and especially young men, would benefit from further help in learning how to negotiate their use.

Integrating education about contraception into a wider programme of personal relationships and self-awareness would identify it with communication and social skills. Bremner and Hillin (1993) point out that if this were to begin at an early age then it would be possible to establish an understanding of the nature of affection and relationships before embarking on the negative connotations of sex such as disease and unwanted pregnancy. They also state, however, that a coordinated and long-term approach such as this is rare and that 'unplanned interventions are common'.

The Children Act makes it clear that a social services department or other caring agency has a duty to cover this aspect of a looked after young person's education. But just as young people have a right to sex education, carers and social workers should be entitled to guidelines, policy statements, training and support in connection with its delivery, and these were regularly absent.

5   Future aspirations

We have seen how the experiences of young people in public care have differed from those in the comparator sample in respect of the way they have been parented, their relationships with adults, peers and partners, their sex education and their attitude towards sex and relationships. In this chapter we attempt to explore to what extent these experiences might affect their views of and aspirations for the future.

One possible reason advanced for young people in general choosing to become parents at an early age is the lack of attractive alternatives available to them. This might be especially true of those looked after whose education has been disrupted and whose employment prospects might look bleak. Thus, for some, pregnancy may be a considered option, or at least *an* option when no others present themselves. The assumption of a 'deficit model' of teenage parenthood is not always appropriate. Two 17-year-old mothers, both of whom had suffered highly disruptive and abusive childhoods and were now bringing up children alone, also drew attention to the fact that they were losing nothing, particularly in respect of their childhood.

'They always bring up your lost childhood. For me, I didn't have a childhood in the first place.'

'I mean, you lose your childhood but I never had much anyway so there isn't really much to lose.'

However, the information obtained from the young mothers in component 1 indicates that many did have aims for the future above and beyond parenthood and that becoming pregnant was in many cases an interference in their plans. But the majority were of the opinion that, although they had not intended to have the baby, they were not going to allow it, and in some cases already had not allowed it, to prevent them achieving at least some of their ambitions.

'I didn't expect it all to come so soon. I had plans for things I was doing, going to college, carrying on education, get a career and all the rest of it. It's not all gone to plan ... I'm not letting it change too much ... But if I'd thought of having children, it would've been a lot later on, when I'd done everything I wanted to do. When I'd come to the end of my plan, that probably would've been in the next one.' (*17-year-old, pregnant, continuing in education*)

'I just wanted to get a career and sort my life out before getting pregnant, but I put it there so I've got to get rid of the problem ... I still want to have a career. I'd still like to work in the prison service. It's just a question of trying to balance it all out.' (*17-year-old, pregnant*)

'I did want to go and work for the social services or somewhere around that area but, I mean, I can do it while she is at school.' (*19-year-old with child aged one and a half*)

'I don't feel as though I've missed out on anything because of having K apart from going to college. I will get the qualifications but I've no idea what I'm going to do with them after that. I don't think K has really made much difference to any of that.' (*16-year-old with child aged one, attending college, taking 'A' levels*)

'I had plans but there is nothing that I can't go ahead with. The way I see it, something else has come into my life and it is my duty to look after her ... I would have been an interior designer, hopefully.' (*17-year-old with child aged seven months, intending to resume education*)

'I would've been at college now but I'll have to go next year and I think I'll be more determined now because I've got C and I'll have to provide money for him.' (*16-year-old with child aged two months*)

'I wanted to stop at the children's home for a while, get my own bedroom, go to college and settle down but it worked out differently. I still want to be somebody. I would like to go to university and get a degree but not yet.' (*16-year-old with child aged 16 months, passed GCSEs when already had the baby*)

How young people see their future

In component 2 the presence of the school sample allowed us to compare the aims and expectations for the future of a looked after sample with those of young people not looked after. We look first at their general expectations and then at those that relate specifically to education, employment and relationships.

The majority of respondents in both samples did not agree with the statement that 'young people today have a good future to look forward to'. Girls in both samples were most likely to disagree with the statement while the highest level of agreement came from the boys in the school sample (Table A.1, Appendix B).

For looked after young people an important aspect of their lives is the degree of control that they have over it. Both samples were asked in the questionnaire whether they felt they had been involved in the plans and decisions made about their lives. Of those looked after 36 per cent said they had been involved in all of them but only a quarter of girls compared with nearly half the boys considered this to be the case. Girls were much more likely to think that they had been involved in *some* rather than all of them, while the proportions thinking that they had not been involved at all (12.5 per cent) differed very little according to gender. In the school sample the proportion who felt they had not been involved was very similar to that in the looked after sample. The main difference lay in the fact that over half (and 60 per cent of boys) felt that they had been involved in *all* of the decisions and plans.

Thus, compared with their non-looked after peers, young people in public care are less used to being consulted about what will happen to them. For example, when routinely asked in interviews how long they would be remaining in their current placement the vast majority said they did not know. They have little experience of planning for the future and very few examples of how this is effectively accomplished. When speaking generally about their experiences of care, many of them with considerable indignation, referred to the manner in which decisions about their accommodation were made: short-term decisions at short notice, without consultation and with no respect for their views.

'I'd been with a short-term foster carer. It was for four years but it was supposed to be short term.' (*Female*)

'I went to look at a placement down there in November, early December, but I couldn't go down there because of the funding, so I come here instead ... everything was going on fine but they didn't have enough funding so ...' (*Female*)

'I didn't know whether I was going to be in one place for five minutes or a couple of days or a week or even a month. I just got moved around so many times. (*Female*)

'It was only six months temporary, so they could find me another placement. In the end I stayed 12 months.' (*Male*)

In a group discussion two young people explained their attitude and the effect on them of decisions made in this way.

'I think social services just like to move you around ...'
'It is hard to trust people cos I was told I was only going to be in, come in here for a couple, three days yes. I was in here for a week, then they told

me I'd be here for two weeks, it just goes on and on, and I've been here nearly seven months now. '

'They think it's for your own benefit.'

(Mixed gender looked after group)

In another conversation between two young people they attempted to understand the theory behind the practice.

'You know what they did to me? At X House they said to me they weren't going to move me for a quite a long time – I were here two days after.'
'I were only meant to be in X House for a week, I was there for over a month.'
Why do you think that is? (*Researcher*)
'They don't know, but they like you to think that they do, do you know what I mean? B (a carer) from X House told me that they don't know themselves but they want you to feel secure.'
'They just don't want you to run away and that. They know you're going to be in that home a certain amount of time but they don't want you to run away so they won't tell you. They just make excuses about "Oh, we haven't sorted it out yet".'
Would you rather be told that they didn't know? (*Researcher*)
'I'd rather they told you the truth instead of lying to you ... They think you're stupid.'
'It's best that you know. I mean, it's your life, you need to know. It's your right, do you know what I mean?'
'You need to know what's going on.'
'No one has the right to lie to you about what's going to happen ... It's not staff, it's social workers that have got to be moving you here there and everywhere. So we should know.'
'They just think it's easy for us.'
'They do, don't they?'
'They just think, "Oh, they don't give a shit if they move or not", but we do.'
'Course you do, it's where you're going to be living.'
'... but they decide things for you.'

The undesirability of this practice and the adverse effect on children and young people have been highlighted recently (House of Commons, 1998). One consequence for the young people in our sample was the development of a tendency to live for the day. When asked whether they worried about the future they often replied in the following terms:

'I definitely don't (worry about the future). If it happens, it happens. If it don't, it don't.' (*Male*)

'If it happens, it happens. Whatever, I don't really mind.' (*Female*)

'I mean, I don't usually think that far ahead. If anything I think a couple of days ahead; plan out my day and that's it. If I get to the day and do the things I'm most pleased but if I don't, I don't … Mmm. I've always thought like that … I mean, if you don't do it, you don't do it. I mean, some things you don't get to do, some things you do.' (*Female*)

Many of those who made this type of comment indicated that they were adopting a philosophical attitude to the future. Of greater potential concern is the relatively large number who accompanied this with a statement to the effect that they were unsure of their future existence, not *what* they would be doing.

'I just look to the present and I just take the future as it comes, cos I find you don't know what to expect in the future, cos for all we know, tomorrow we could be dead. What's the point of planning your future? Just take the future as it comes, like.' (*Female*)

'Where am I going to be in five years from now? Am I going to be dead or am I still going to be alive …' (*Male*)

'And then in the year 2000 I don't know what I'll be doing, if I'm still around by then.' (*Female*)

This fatalistic attitude, which in many cases also applied to their views about pregnancy ('If they get pregnant, they get pregnant, you know what I mean' – *Male*), was noticeably absent in the school sample. However, when asked whether they had plans for the future, the majority of the looked after young people replied that they did. More in the looked after sample than in the school sample claimed to have definite rather than vague ideas, although we might, on the basis of the evidence from component 1 discussed later in this chapter, question to what extent these were realistic.

Respondents to the component 2 questionnaire were asked to select from a list of seven options which they would like to be doing in four years' time. In retrospect it might seem unrealistic to have asked them to have ideas about their future four years' hence when in many cases they do not know where they will be living tomorrow and consequently some of the results may be subject to idealisation.

The results are set out in Table 5.1. In the looked after sample, most respondents wanted to be in a secure job and there was no gender difference. About three quarters said that in four years' time they would like either to be doing some form of training or be at college or university, a surprisingly high proportion in view of their stated dislike of school and their willingness to absent themselves whenever possible: 44 per cent admitted that they skipped school whenever they had the chance. Many more girls than boys wanted to be in further education (83 per cent of girls

Table 5.1   In four years' time would like to ...

	Looked after (%)			School (%)		
	Total	Male	Female	Total	Male	Female
Be still living in the town or place where currently living	56	51	62*	62	74*	46
Be in a secure job	92	92	92	77.5	84.5	68
Be in a steady relationship with someone	88.5	87.5	90	86	84	89
Be at college or university (or about to go)	72	62	83	70	67	73
Have at least one child	51*	55*	47*	24	30	17
Be doing some form of training	76	65	85	77	81*	71
Be married or living with a boyfriend or girlfriend	65*	80*	48	40	42	38

*Significant difference from comparative samples.

compared with 62 per cent of boys) or in some form of training (85 per cent of girls and 65 per cent of boys). In response to a subsequent question nearly three quarters of the looked after girls had expressed agreement with the statement that 'Having a job is the best way for a woman to be an independent person', a proportion higher than that of the boys and marginally higher than that of the girls in the school sample. Possibly with this in mind they considered that education represented the first step on that route to independence. Fewer school sample respondents expressed a preference for being in a secure job or in education or training. As in the looked after sample, more girls than boys opted for further or higher education but, conversely, more boys than girls opted for training, which was not the case in the looked after sample.

For the school sample, a greater priority than being in employment or education was being in a steady relationship and more girls than boys wanted this, although the difference was only slight. Although it seemed not to be so important for the young people in public care, nevertheless *a larger percentage* of them than in the school sample aspired to a steady relationship (88.5 per cent) with little difference according to gender. But many more looked after boys than girls (80 per cent as opposed to 48 per cent) also said that they would like to be married or living with a partner. In addition more boys than girls said that they would like to have at least one child by then (55 per cent of boys and 47 per cent of girls) The proportions were substantially, and in most cases also significantly, higher than those found among the school sample. As in the looked after sample, more boys than girls wanted to have child and be married or cohabiting.

Those in the looked after sample were less likely than young people in the school sample to want to remain in the town or place where they currently lived. In the looked after sample more girls than boys wanted to stay put while in the school sample the reverse applied, with nearly three quarters of the boys wanting to remain in their home town.

Education

As we see from replies to the question above, the young people in both samples set considerable store by continuing their education. But more than half of those looked after had previously stated that they did not like school and we have already noted above the extent to which they do not attend whenever they have the opportunity.

The frequent and unscheduled changes of placement which they suffer can also lead to disrupted education, or even its premature termination, for the reasons set out below by two young people.

'And every time you move somewhere, you know, like into another foster parent you have to move schools, and it just does your head in. You just don't know what's going on. And if you're doing your GCSEs, like I were gonna do, I just got moved and then I had to start another school.'
'And they're all doing different work.'
'Yeah. I just did all this work what they were doing and I just shot through it all and the teacher said, "Do something else." And I said, "What the fuck do I do? I've finished it." I'm just going on my GCSEs and he says, "We're not entering you for GCSEs for another year." So I said, "Fuck it" and I walked out of the class and never went back.'
'It's, like, all the work they're doing now at (current school), I've done it already.'
'Yeah, you do everything, don't you and then you've got to go back and do it again.'
'That always seems to happen. Wherever I've gone, I've always done it before at another school. So it's piss easy and when it's so easy I just get bored. And then when it's too hard I get bored!'

Another young woman, who had experienced 16 foster placements, described the disruption and disorientation associated with having to go to a new school at the same time as adjusting to a new placement:

'It makes it harder for the first two weeks or something, because you're all confused. You've got to travel to school or something, you probably have to leave school earlier to get home, to find your way home.' (*Female*)

Several of the young people interviewed in component 2 had not changed schools with each placement. While the continuity was a bonus, the main disadvantage lay in the amount of time spent travelling to and from school, particularly for those living in a large city. They often recounted how the journey required them to travel to the opposite side of the city, a journey that typically took over an hour. One young man explained that the formidable nature of the journey frequently influenced his decision about whether he would go to school.

> 'Cause, don't know, I just, my school is ages away and I just, you know what I mean – sometimes I wake up and I think, "Oh, I don't want to go to school today" and I just don't go.' (*Male*)

There were also those who disliked going to school because they suffered taunts about being in the care system.

> 'Like just when I'm at college, like people say, "What's it like, being in care?" I just, like, turned round to this bloke, R, and I says, "I don't give a shit what it's like because I'm coming out and I don't really want to talk about it so shut that up" ... Some people just like ask and ask and ask and, like, some people are, like, taking the piss.' (*Male*)

And there were also those who were bullied to the extent that they became suicidal:

> 'I was taking pills because I was too scared to go back into school.' (*Female*)

There were also those whose background or lack of current support meant that persisting in education was difficult. One young man pointed out that he had been disadvantaged from the start by his parents:

> 'When you don't go to school and those times you think it's fun but now I wish I had done a lot more at school. I wished I was in a better environment when I first started school ... Like my family background and that. It would have helped me.' (*Male*)

And one young woman explained how her foster carers booked a family foreign holiday for the two-week period when she should have been taking public exams:

> 'All the teachers were saying, "You should stop here and do your exams, you can go on holiday any time" and I said, "I'm not changing it, I'm going on holiday".' (*Female*)

A further complication is that some young women had used school as an escape from abuse at home, spending excessively long hours there. Once removed from the abuse they no longer had the incentive to be at school: even more importantly, school, and abuse might be linked in their mind.

> 'When I lived with me dad I used to go to school like every day because I was scared of going home and getting clattered. So I were, like, in school all day every day, you know. But I were just scared all the time, I didn't want to go home after school and stuff like that. Then I didn't go home so that made me dad mad and then I'd get clattered even more.' (*Female*)

'When I was at home I'd get up at half five, and leave school for ten to seven, just to get out, so that school was like a relief from home ... it's getting a bit boring now, school, but I still like it.' (*Female*)

Consequently, taking into account their experiences and difficulties associated with education, it is surprising that so many expressed a desire to remain in the educational system. This was, however, not borne out in the interviews with this sample where most were more concerned about getting a job than getting qualifications.

One young woman who had earlier spelt out the extent to which her education had suffered over the years expressed a desire to be either a lawyer or a police officer but was opting for the latter because:

'One, I don't have to spend five years or so in law school and, secondly, I can get the grades for a police officer much more easily.'

In the rare cases where some ambition for further education had been formulated it was subject to sabotage from areas beyond those associated with money which respondents in the school sample had articulated.

'Learning is interesting, I want to learn, it's just remembering what you learn, I sometimes have trouble with that, because of my surroundings here, everything's getting on my nerves, the isolation, it all builds up and I can't concentrate, but you just make yourself concentrate and eventually it does work.'
What do your family think about your wanting to go on to university? Will they support you? (*Researcher*)
'Probably my aunt and uncle would like me to, I'm not sure about my mum and everybody there, whether they would support me, I don't know.' (*Male*)

In contrast to the above, most of those in the school sample said they wanted to stay on at school until they were 18 and most wanted to continue their education beyond. While many of them had set their sights on a career which required education to degree level, others were aiming at further education courses leading to vocational work. Only one young man in the school interview sample intended to leave school at the age of 16. Many background variables, including the ethos of the schools and socioeconomic factors which were not controlled for, could jointly and severally account for their attitude towards higher education.

It is possible that the high level of agreement of the looked after young people with the question about continuing education may be connected to giving an answer they considered likely to suit or impress the researcher or to thinking that they *would* like to do this (which is what the question asked) while not pausing to consider the implications. This was, to some extent, true of the mothers in component 1. Many of those who had finished their education before the minimum leaving age spoke of 'going to college' as their next step. Most seemed oblivious to the fact that attending school or college with a baby was considerably harder than doing so without one – and they had not always had distinguished attendance records in the past.

Only three young women in component 1 were attending college and taking higher qualifications at the time of the interview. Chapter 9 addresses some of the difficulties faced by pregnant young women and young mothers in respect of their education.

Although social workers who were interviewed in our study were supportive of the young women being in or returning to education, only one specifically mentioned it as her responsibility and stressed the future implications:

> 'I have a duty to see that they get some education and it's an important aspect of their life. They'll need it in the future if they want to get a job.'

In the component 2 vignettes about the young couple (see Table A.2, Appendix B), respondents were asked to decide what the 15-year-old girl should do about her education once she became pregnant. There were many similarities between the samples in the level of responses but the main difference lay in the greater proportion of school sample respondents suggesting that she should continue her education because she would need qualifications to obtain a good job later (69 per cent as opposed to 54 per cent of the looked after sample). School sample boys were most in favour of this. More of them than in the looked after sample also advocated her leaving school straightaway. Among the girls the most favoured option was to seek admission to the school for pregnant schoolgirls. More of the school sample girls (81 per cent) than the looked after girls (62 per cent) advocated this. This also received support from 63 per cent of the looked after boys.

Employment

Component 2 questionnaire respondents were asked whether they currently had a part-time job. Those who did were confined primarily to the school sample where 42 had a job of some sort compared with 12 in the looked after sample. The usual jobs were babysitting, shop work, cafe, bar or hotel work, and paper rounds. In the looked after sample, seven of the 12 who said they had a job did not specify what it was. Some in the school sample, especially boys, reported in interviews that a friend of their father had been responsible for giving them employment:

> 'Because, like, I'm actually working for my dad's friend, my mechanic job. He's an engineer and he does it on the side.'

His companion in this discussion highlighted the importance of having connections in obtaining full-time employment in the future:

'It's, like, if you know a lot of people you can get jobs in places because you know people, if you've got lots of friends and that.'

This was not an avenue open to many looked after young people who had no, few or unsatisfactory dealings with their father.

Having a job, or specifically having a good job, was often cited by those in both samples in interviews as something they worried most about as regards the future.

'Having a good job, and money.'

'You need a job to support yourself and then support a family. It's the key to a lot of things.'

(School sample, males)

The school sample respondents invariably had already formulated an idea of the type of work they would do in the future. For the boys this usually involved working in information technology or mechanical engineering. For girls who intended to continue into higher education subsequent career options included the legal profession, astronomy, teaching and youth work, and for those not intending to pursue their education a caring profession had most appeal.

The young people interviewed in the looked after sample were more vague than those in the school sample about their aspirations and tended to tie them to their current recreational pursuits. Many of the young men aspired to 'doing something with computers' or being professional footballers, acknowledging that this was a pipe dream but failing to put a more realistic ambition in place.

'I'd like to be a footballer.'

A professional footballer? (*Researcher*)

'But I'll never make that ... I can play football but I'm not anything special. I'm more of a watcher – let them do all the work.'

So if you can't be a professional footballer what else might you do? (*Researcher*)

'Listen to music – except you don't get paid for that.'

Another 15-year-old male with little musical success to date and even less encouragement entertained ambitions to become a rock star:

'I'll make it alone or I'll make it in a band but I'm going to make it.'

The young women were equally unsure, often saying they wanted to work with children but having no information about what would be involved in the way of training.

What do you have to do for training to be a nursery teacher? (*Researcher*)

'I don't know.'

So nobody's told you what it needs? (*Researcher*)
'No.'
Do you think it'll be difficult? (*Researcher*)
'Not really, cos I already know how to handle kids ... I've got three little nieces.'

Questionnaire respondents were also asked to consider which, if any, of a range of statements might apply to their not getting job they wanted in the future (Table 5.2). The two groups identified similar obstacles to obtaining employment, such as lack of qualifications and training and a shortage of jobs. While the looked after boys were more aware than the girls of the potential lack of jobs and of their own qualifications, the girls were more conscious of their own lack of experience. As we have seen, very few looked after girls had any form of part-time employment. In the school sample, girls appeared to be much more conscious than either their male peers, or the looked after girls, that they may be held back by employment or educational factors both within and outside their control.

Crucially, 50 per cent of those in public care compared with only 9 per cent of the comparator group envisaged that their background would have a detrimental effect on their obtaining a job they would like, and 44 per cent, compared with 12 per cent of those not in public care, also thought that their employment prospects would be damaged through having been in trouble with the law.

Table 5.2   Factors that young people thought might stop them getting a job they would like in the future

	Looked after (%)			School (%)		
	Total	Male	Female	Total	Male	Female
You won't want to move away from this area	24	23.5	25	24	24	23
Your background will be a disadvantage	50*	49*	50*	9	10	8.5
There aren't enough jobs available	44	49	38.5	53	49	57*
You won't have enough qualifications or training	49.5	53*	46	41	36	47
You may already have a child	22	14	31*	16	17	15
Your family will want you to stay at home	18	22	15	18	17	19
You won't have the experience	36	27.5	44	27	19	38
You may have been in trouble with the law	44*	51*	36.5*	16	17	15
Some other reason	8	8	8	12	8.5	17

*Significant difference from comparative samples.

While a greater proportion of boys than girls in public care were concerned about the potential effect of criminal activities, the girls were significantly more likely than the boys, and significantly more likely than the girls in the comparator sample, to state that already having a child might thwart their employment ambitions. Nearly a third of them thought this might be so.

Thus we can see that looked after young people were highly conscious of the fact that both their background and their behaviour, including becoming pregnant, had the potential to affect their employment prospects. While just as concerned as their non-looked after peers about a lack of jobs, qualifications and training, and in some cases even more so, they had other anxieties that weighed more heavily.

The majority of the young mothers in component 1 were not in employment outside the home. Those who were in some form of paid work were engaged in unskilled part-time work. Most of them had intentions to take up paid work as soon as they could, mainly out of a determination not to stay 'on the social'. Only one had, according to her carer, no intention of gaining employment. Her bitterness and resentment at having been looked after since early childhood and having suffered a number of unhappy placements had affected her attitude towards the future:

'B has no interest at all in employment, to be honest with you. She's said she's no interest – she's not going to work. "The state's going to keep me for the rest of my life." Which is sad really. She's got this thing: "Well, you put me in care, you can look after me now".'

In contrast another carer described the attitude of a 17-year-old mother:

'She's got this child: all right she knows it was a mistake, but it's there ... She will be hoping that, by finishing the course off, some day she will be able to get herself in some form of employment so that she would then be able to keep the child.'

Furstenburg, Brooks-Gunn and Morgan (1987) indicate on the basis of a longitudinal study that most young mothers do not rely on welfare payments indefinitely and clearly it was not the intention of the vast majority of these young women to do so. This calls into question one of the reasons put forward by Hudson and Ineichen (1991) as to why young women become pregnant (see Chapter 6).

Their choice of future employment typically involved work in a caring profession: working with animals, children and the elderly were most strongly favoured and many young women had had work experience with their chosen group. Their sense of injustice at what had happened to them in the past prompted desires to help others in the future. Frequently they expressed a desire to take up work with a social services department either in residential child care or as a social worker. One young woman recounted her reasons:

I want to be a social worker, I've really set my heart on it ... Because the life that I've had, by my teenage age, I think I understand kids more. You know, like, when I'm older, because I've been there and done that, do you get what I mean? A lot of social workers ... like, when they tell me where they live and their mum lives and I'm thinking they've come from a nice, posh home and their mum's like a such and such, something good. I'm thinking when they're talking to you, "They don't know what the hell they're talking about." ... When I first went to social services like, I got in contact with social services, my mum got in touch with social services, when I spoke to them I didn't really want to talk to them because I knew that they didn't know what I was going through ... because they hadn't experienced it. And like, I know, right, if a social worker says to me, "Well, I got pregnant at 15 as well," I'd want to listen, I'd *want* to listen. And I'd probably get on more with that social worker, I'd want to listen to her. She'd go, "And I didn't get on with my mum" and whatever, and I'd want to listen. But all the social workers don't, most of them. Because they'd probably listen to me more, knowing that I've experienced it ... Because I know that they haven't been through nothing. They've come from a good home or whatever.' (*15-year-old with three-month-old baby*)

Among the young mothers in component 1, those who had continued or were continuing their education were usually realistic about what they needed to achieve to follow their chosen career. One young woman remained in education, gaining qualifications, simply because she was too young at 17 to pursue her career, for which she did not need the qualifications. Such awareness and application were rare: much more common was a picture of education that had been disrupted and ended prematurely accompanied by an ambition to be a social worker, a gynaecologist or a psychiatrist. This might call into question whether such plans were formulated when it was too late to achieve them. If not, then the unfortunate, and the saddest, aspect was the extent to which the young women were unaware of what was involved in achieving their goals. It is hard to imagine that their future ambitions had not been discussed with their social worker and surprising that they had not been given reliable information on courses of study leading to required qualifications. It seemed to be yet another area of their lives where these young women were likely to fail.

Relationships and partners

While family life and sexual relationships are discussed in greater detail in Chapters 2 and 3, in this section we examine young people's intentions and aspirations for the future as regards partnerships, marriage and parenthood.

The young mothers and mothers-to-be in component 1 were predominantly living alone. Although some had been in relationships with the father of the child, these had usually not endured and others which did exist were reportedly not secure. Nevertheless the majority did aspire to partnership, and preferably marriage, at some point in the future. When asked how they saw their lives in three years' time virtually all the replies from the young women included a husband or partner, as this example illustrates:

'I don't have a picture of what I would like it to be. I'm quite happy like this ... I would like to eventually settle down and have another baby with someone who maybe I could stay with and be a proper family – the other parent there as well. You can't guarantee things are going to work out all the time but that would be nice, to be sharing it with somebody else and not just on your own. I don't want to be on my own for the rest of my life.' (*19-year-old with child of 18 months*)

We have already seen above that the hopes for the future of most component 2 respondents encompassed being in a steady relationship by the time they were 19 or 20. Although slightly more girls than boys indicated this, more boys than girls wanted to be living with or married to a partner. As many as three quarters of the looked after boys agreed that they would like this to happen in four years' time, significantly more than both looked after girls and school sample boys (see Table 5.1).

In response to a further question, just over half the school sample thought that they would get married, compared with just over one third of the looked after sample. In both samples more boys than girls thought they would, the gender difference being particularly marked in the school sample. As a whole young people in the looked after sample were much more likely to reply that they *might* marry. Forty-three per cent overall replied in this way with no difference according to gender. But a quarter of the looked after girls did not intend to marry at all. None of the school sample and very few of the looked after sample considered that they would marry only if they had children.

The mean for what they considered the ideal age for people (not necessarily themselves) to get married lay between 20 and 21 although the age most commonly cited by all the girls was 18. For boys in the school sample it was 21 and for those in the looked after sample it was 20. However, the number of responses to this question was low as the majority thought there was no 'ideal' age to marry.

Making plans for the future does not come easily to young people looked after and this was borne out in relation to this question about marriage in the qualitative part of component 2. When asked whether they thought they would marry, one young man in a group discussion exclaimed, 'I ain't even thought about what I'm gonna do tomorrow, never mind marrying somebody!'.

As we have noted, the prospect of having a child in four years' time appealed more to boys than to girls and especially those looked after. Nevertheless the interview data showed that most young people in both samples thought that they would become a parent at some point. There were exceptions to this in both samples but these rested mainly with looked after boys and school sample girls. In the former case, when the topic of being a parent was introduced into a discussion one young man replied succinctly 'Oh well fuck that. I ain't gonna be a parent.' However, further conversation led him to state, 'I don't know about ever, but I just don't know, I ain't thought about that yet'.

Some school sample girls expressed reservations because they professed not to like children or because they did not want to give birth:

'The only thing that puts me a bit off having children, I know it sounds stupid, but it's the pain. I haven't got a very big pain threshold.'

'I just don't want to give birth to them. I want to wait till they've invented a drug so you don't actually have to give birth.'

This was not the case with the looked after girls, who either had not considered the matter or were not disturbed at the prospect. No young women cited factors connected to career advancement for women or the difficulty of combining material success with the needs of children as reasons for not having children.

The component 2 quantitative data included young people's opinions of the 'best age' to start having children. About one quarter of each sample thought that there was no ideal age, but those who replied stated that, on average, it was best to start a family at 21 or 22, although the most common age quoted was 20. Hope and Sharland (1997) quoted the most common age as between 22 and 23.

This was slightly at odds with statements from those who had said that they would like to have a child when they were 19 or 20 (that is in four years' time) and with the interview data. In interviews the majority thought that they would like to have their first child when they were in their mid-20s or, for some of the school sample, in their late-20s. However, while the former question was phrased in general terms, the discussion in the interviews revolved round them personally, and in this respect they may have considered themselves delaying the start of their family. Twenty-five is probably an age sufficiently far removed from their own to allow them to have achieved, in their minds, all that they wish to. Even those in the school sample who were intending to go on to higher education did not appear to consider that four years after qualifying was a relatively short period of time. There was considerable discussion around this topic in the interviews:

'About late 20s to middle 30s ... Because I want to have some fun when I'm younger.'

And do you think fun ends when you have children? (*Researcher*)
'Depends on what sort of fun you mean. There's fun when you go to nightclubs and it will end then, you know, but if you mean fun staying in and watching football and having a few beers or something, that'll be all right.' (*Male looked after*)

'Once I got picked up on a job and I've got good money and I've got a girlfriend or whatever, then I've decide ... 25, sort of. I just want to enjoy my life as much as I can.' (*Male looked after*)

'I won't have them until I've got a really stable career.' (*Female looked after*)

'Well not before I'm, like, 25 ... That's it. I know that from me mum. She's got four, there's four of us altogether now. And her whole life's revolved around babies ... I want my life to happen.' (*Female looked after*)

'About 27. Get set up first ... it's the right time. More mature.'
'Like (earlier) you want to go out with your friends and go to pubs and that sort of thing.'

(*Mixed school group*)

'I guess about 26 ... I'd like to have a good career and know I'd be stable and staying in the relationship as well ... yeah, I'd like the dad to be part of it. If there's no love there, it won't happen will it?'
'... about 20, 20–22 and the relationship should be good because you can't really cope on your own, going out to work and getting all the money to clothe them and feed them and the mortgage and that, so you need to be in a relationship and a good job.'

(*Females, school sample*)

The majority intended becoming parents within a marriage or a steady relationship and beginning parenthood as a lone mother was rejected by most girls. However, the fatalistic acceptance which we noted earlier was also evident here: one young woman remarked, 'I wouldn't want to be a single parent but if it happens, it happens.'

Summary points

All young people in both samples of component 2 considered that employment was the most important aspect of their future but all could foresee obstacles to their obtaining a job that they would like. These included a shortage of jobs, lack of qualifications and lack of experience. However, a significant difference between the two samples was that the looked after young people, and especially the boys, also considered that their background and their having committed a criminal offence would be equally instrumental in their not gaining a desired job. And a substantial proportion of looked after girls thought that already having a child would be an obstacle for them.

The majority aspired to being in a permanent relationship and having children at some time in the future. When asked to consider the future in four years' time (when they were 19 or 20), all thought that being in a steady relationship was important to them but many more of the looked after young people, and among them more boys than girls, wanted to be married or cohabiting *and* to have a child by then.

The young mothers in component 1 who were mainly without a partner at the time of interview envisaged their future in terms of marriage or cohabitation rather than lone parenthood. They were also keen to be self-supporting and not dependent on welfare benefits indefinitely, although sometimes they had aspirations to employment that could not realistically be achieved.

Young people looked after both see and plan for the future differently from those who are not looked after. Their experience of the future is typically a series of short-term interventions based on decisions made by other people. Consequently they have a fatalistic acceptance of events coupled with a fore-shortened view of the future and operate on a time scale that precludes looking at a period years hence:

> 'You don't know what you're gonna do tomorrow, do you, or the rest of your life ... It's like, day before yesterday seems like last week, you know what I mean?'

Often in calculating ages they make mistakes that appear to relate more to concepts of time than to basic errors of mental arithmetic. Thus, having a child at 15 meant you would be 50 when it was 18; or 25 was a good age for having children because it is 'an inbetween age, between 24 and 50 really'.

Therefore in interpreting their responses it should be remembered that they are probably not seeing the future as clearly as young people in the school sample nor do they necessarily have confidence in achieving the things to which they aspire. Moreover, it is clear from their responses that early partnership and parenthood have a stronger attraction for young people in public care than for those who are not, and that they are aware that their experience of having been in public care may be an obstacle to their achieving what they wish.

6   Pregnancy and decision making

This chapter first explores the views of young people on why teenagers become pregnant. It then looks at reactions of looked after young people once a pregnancy is discovered, how they reach decisions about whether to continue with the pregnancy, and the support they receive in making such a decision. This latter section is based mainly on the findings from component 1 of the study, the qualitative interviews with mothers and mothers-to-be and with social workers and carers. Where possible, comparisons are made with their peers in the wider community, based on other research evidence.

Teenage conceptions and maternities

In 1996 just over 94,000 young women under 20 in England and Wales became pregnant, slightly over half of whom were 'older' teenage mothers (aged 18 or 19) and fewer than 10 per cent (8800) were under 16. Wellings and others (1994) concluded that fewer than 10 per cent of the British population was at risk of an unintended pregnancy while data from the 1993 General Household Survey (Office of Population Censuses and Surveys, 1995) suggested that this was as low as 3 per cent. However, this proportion is concentrated in the youngest age groups (Cartwright, 1988). Furthermore the implications of an unplanned pregnancy for younger women may be far greater than for older women. Women in the older age groups might not have planned a pregnancy at that particular time but might find it easier to reconcile this into their pattern of life, with the result that such a pregnancy, while initially unplanned, might not be unwanted. For young women who are being or have recently been looked after, adjusting to an unplanned pregnancy is not an easy task, particularly in practical terms.

Yet many of them choose to carry the baby to term. We have already noted the link between low rates of teenage abortion and low socio-economic group. Other factors that have been documented as affecting why a young woman would choose to seek a termination of a pregnancy are social and family pressures, the age of the young woman and the nature of her relationship with the baby's father (Houghton, 1994). But little is known about the method by which young women actually reach the decision about whether to continue or terminate a pregnancy (Allen and Bourke Dowling, 1998). Understanding why young women become pregnant and then carry the baby to term is important in determining what action might be taken to reduce either conceptions or maternities that are unplanned.

Hudson and Ineichen (1991, pp. 42–46) advance 18 reasons why adolescents choose to carry the baby to term, amongst which are:

- genuine ignorance of the pregnancy;
- rebellion against parents;
- an object to love;
- to keep the father;
- to achieve adult status;
- to confirm a prophesy that they are 'a bad lot';
- to gain access to housing;
- disaffection from school;
- pressure from a boyfriend to keep the child;
- mistakes and poor advice about abortion;
- fatalistic acceptance.

More than 30 years ago the observation was made in respect of teenage mothers that:

> They hoped to satisfy their wish to feel needed, loved and good, not only in the arms of their boy friends but also through their babies' need and love of them. (Gough, 1964)

However, on the basis of her interviews with young mothers Burghes (1995, p. 41) comments that 'the attitudes that persuaded the mothers to keep their babies were complex and difficult to disentangle' and that decisions to see the pregnancy through were not taken lightly.

Reasons for early parenthood: the views of young people

It was clear that the young people in both components of our research did not advocate having children during adolescence, irrespective of whether they had done so themselves. Since the views of adults about why young people do so are frequently aired, we were keen to explore the views of teenagers themselves on this topic, and the possible reasons for teenagers becoming pregnant was a focal point of both the quantitative and qualitative sections of component 2. The findings from these confirm some of the findings from component 1 and contradict others, as might be expected since these (component 2) are based on supposition of others' motives while the former (component 1) represent the explanation of those who became pregnant.

The questionnaire contained a list of ten possible reasons why teenagers become pregnant with which respondents were asked to indicate their agreement or disagreement. Although the statements were listed in random order on the questionnaire, they belonged in three distinct categories relating to: pressure to have sex; prevention of pregnancy; and emotional influences. The results are set out in Table 6.1.

If the statements are ranked according to the percentage agreeing with each one, then in the view of the looked after young people the main reasons for teenagers becoming pregnant were: teenagers don't think they will get pregnant (prevention); teenagers want something to love (emotional response); the girl wants a baby (emotional response); teenagers are careless (prevention); and boys pressurise girls into having sex (pressure). As we see, these responses cover all three categories. The same five statements featured in the top responses from the school sample but were differently ranked. While 'teenagers don't think they will get pregnant' was the statement most frequently agreed with, this was followed by 'teenagers are careless' (both prevention), then 'boys pressurise girls', 'teenagers want something to love' and 'the girl wants a baby'. The proportions agreeing with the last two (emotional reasons) were far lower than among the looked after sample.

If we examine responses according to the three categories we see that there are similarities between the samples in respect of their views about

Table 6.1 Do you think that teenage pregnancies happen for any of the following reasons?

	Looked after (%)			School (%)		
	Total	Male	Female	Total	Male	Female
Teenagers don't think they will be pregnant	85	87	83	81.5	77	86
Teenagers are careless	71	68	73*	62.5	67	57
Teenagers don't know how to use contraception	37	36	37	47	50	44
Teenagers don't know where to get contraception	26	21	30	34	37*	30
Boys pressurise girls into having sex	56	34	76	61	48*	75
Girls pressurise boys into having sex	33	49*	18	24	25	23
Teenagers want something to love	79*	74*	84*	52	44	59.5
The girl wants a baby	72*	71*	72*	50.5	55	45
The boy wants a baby	26	27	24	30	44*	15
Girls want to trap their boyfriends	51*	53	49*	35	39	31

*Significant difference from comparative samples.

prevention but major differences in their views about pressure and emotional reasons.

Prevention

Teenagers believing that they will not become pregnant was the statement most often agreed with by respondents in both samples. Teenagers' carelessness was fourth in the ranking of the looked after sample but second according to the school sample, even though a greater proportion of the looked after sample than the school sample agreed with this. For the statements relating to prevention there was little disparity according to gender and where differences were observed (teenagers are careless and teenagers don't know where to get contraception) these were not marked. However, the gender position was reversed according to the sample: among the young people looked after more girls than boys thought that teenagers were both careless and did not know where to get contraception while in the school sample these views were endorsed by more boys than girls.

Thus the samples are similar in their views about the role of prevention and teenagers' personal responsibility in that direction. Fewer than half in either sample, albeit more in the school sample than the looked after sample, thought that lack of knowledge on how to use contraception or where to obtain it were reasons. It may be inferred from these results that teenagers in general, and especially those in public care, are still in need of further persuasion that they might, in fact, become pregnant and that they should be more careful.

Pressure

In both samples pressure from boys to have sex was much more often cited as a reason than pressure from girls. Not surprisingly, significantly more girls than boys thought the former was the case but the difference between the genders was much greater in the looked after sample due to the fact that significantly fewer looked after boys (34 per cent) than their school sample peers (48 per cent) thought that boys put pressure on girls.

In the responses about girls putting pressure on boys there are noteworthy differences. In the school sample only about a quarter of both boys and girls thought that girls put pressure on boys but in the looked after sample *virtually half the male respondents considered that girls pressurise boys into having sex*. In contrast, less than one fifth of the looked after girls thought this was true.

It is difficult to know whether the view of the looked after boys is based on experience or supposition and it would justify further investigation. However, it can be looked at in relation to other questions and in conjunction with information supplied in component 1. In a previous question on the component 2 questionnaire regarding pressure to have a girlfriend, significantly more of the girls in the looked after sample than in the school sample agreed that boys were put under pressure by their girlfriends. In the first component it was reported by the young mothers that early and unwelcome sexual activity did not necessarily create a continuing aversion to it and that, indeed, the opposite effect may occur. It was also reported that looked after young women felt 'better' if they had a sexual relationship. Further, the considerable freedom associated with living in residential care was referred to by respondents in both components. We might conclude, therefore, that this is not a group of young women with a voracious appetite for sexual activity but rather with an ill-conceived idea of the meaning of affection and of its practical demonstration who have the opportunity to engage in sexual activity. What is not clear is the attitude of the young men. We might usefully explore whether they welcome this attention from girls or whether they, in common with many young women, need help to resist such pressure.

Emotional influences

Looking at the emotional considerations among the looked after sample, roughly equal proportions of both genders considered that the boy wants a baby (about one quarter), girls want to trap their boyfriends (about half) and the girl wants a baby (just less than three quarters) were reasons for teenage pregnancies. However, more girls (84 per cent) than boys (74 per cent) thought that teenagers wanting something to love was an issue, and this was the statement most often agreed with by looked after girls.

It is in this category of statements on emotional influences that most differences between the samples occur. While 52 per cent of the school sample thought that teenagers wanting something to love was a reason for pregnancies occurring, in the looked after sample the proportion was 79 per cent. A similarly large gap is observed in the different level of response to 'the girl wants a baby' (44 per cent in the school sample as opposed to 72 per cent in the looked after sample) and in 'girls want to trap their boyfriends' where the respective proportions were 35 and 50.5 per cent. However, more boys in the school sample than in the looked after sample thought that an issue was *the boy* wanting a baby.

Thus, in the case of the looked after sample, it becomes apparent that their attitudes towards early pregnancy are more complex than those of their peers who are not looked after and that emotional considerations have just as big a part to play as those related to pressure or prevention. It would appear that little progress on the practical side can be achieved if the emotional side remains neglected.

However, it is not just looked after young people who raise potential issues of concern. A relatively high proportion of young men in the school sample attributed the fact that the boy wants a baby to the reasons for teenage pregnancy. If this is looked at in conjunction with the responses to the set of questions about future expectations, where, four years' hence, more boys than girls said they wanted to have a child, be living with a partner and remain in the place where they currently live, then it would suggest that there is scope for making young men in general aware of possible alternatives to early domesticity and for examining the range of options open to them.

The reasons for teenage pregnancy were explored further in interviews and discussion groups in component 2. One of the interesting findings from this part of the study is that most young people *did* have a view. Many claimed personal knowledge of someone who had become pregnant at an early age and only one young woman realised that making assumptions was not necessarily safe:

> 'Well some people make the choice but with some people it's an accident and it's hard to tell unless they actually tell you.'

A major difference between some looked after young women and anyone else in component 2 lay in the fact that they alone offered rape as a possible explanation for pregnancy. Otherwise, certain themes were common within the range of views put forward by the young people. The majority in both samples agreed, as they had in the quantitative study, that invincibility and carelessness had a large part to play in the reasons for pregnancy. But deliberate choice also featured in responses.

A group discussion in one children's home produced a range of responses, many of which were echoed by other participants in interviews.

> 'I think most young girls that get pregnant now ... when they get pregnant they get more attention.'
> 'Or girls who are 16 or something and they live in a hostel and they can't get a flat or something and they get pregnant just to get a flat.'
> 'Some get raped.'
> 'Well they do it to keep – if they love someone, but the geezer don't love her, she might have the baby just to attach him to her so she feels he has a need to stay with her.'
> 'Because they don't use protection.'
> (repeating) 'They don't use protection.'
> 'They don't think about the consequences.'
> 'They think it's a good fuck.'
> 'It's a good laugh now, and they don't think about what's going to happen after. They don't think things through.'
>
> *(Mixed group)*

In an individual interview a young woman elaborated further on some of these topics, drawing on her own experience:

'. . . I know a lot of girls that have been in care that have thought it'd be nice to have a baby, but for other reasons as well. Like they think "If I get pregnant when I'm coming up to 16, I won't get shoved in a hostel, I'll get a flat and I'll have all my bills paid for me" and it don't always work out that way. Some girls do it just to get their boyfriends hooked. I mean, I know someone that tried to get herself pregnant cos her boyfriend was gonna leave her – but I wouldn't do it cos you don't know that it would work out and what goes around comes around, and it's not very nice, is it?'

The many references in the interviews with the looked after young people to 'having someone to love' (or to be loved by) confirmed the questionnaire results, as did using pregnancy as a deliberate ploy in order to gain attention, to gain access to housing or to keep a boyfriend. 'Keeping a boyfriend' was mentioned by young people in both samples and possibly more frequently than anticipated by the school sample in view of their responses to the quantitative question. This is another theory often advanced by 'experts' and reiterated in the list supplied by Hudson and Ineichen (1991), but it did not appear to feature in the thinking of the pregnant women and mothers in the component 1 sample, who entertained a very poor view of the young men in their lives. The idea was very effectively scuppered by the comment of one young woman's mother who succinctly remarked that 'Young girls would get pregnant to keep the father, but now they don't because the fathers just bugger off, don't they?'

'To gain access to housing' had been excluded from the list of options in the questionnaire because of its near-mythical status in connection with lone mothers in general but an unexpectedly large number of looked after young people referred to it. However, no-one in the school sample interviews did. This was one of the reasons stated by Hudson and Ineichen for a young woman carrying a baby to term. They claim that 'this stratagem has worked in the past and girls have been able to use the system to their advantage' (p. 44). This is by no means an uncommon view (Speak and others, 1995), but recent research has indicated that in general young women are unaware of their entitlements to both housing and benefits before they become pregnant (Allen and Bourke Dowling, 1998).

Although single young mothers are six times more likely than the general population to live in areas with more than 75 per cent of social housing (Botting, Rosato and Wood, 1998), this must be as much an indication of their inability to move out as their eagerness to move in. Certainly there is no evidence to support the belief that lone parents are housed by local authorities and housing associations at the expense of two-parent families (Institute of Housing, 1993; Burghes, 1995). Wilson (1994, p. 5), in her research for the House of Commons, established that the high proportion of lone parent families living in council accommodation was generally attributed by housing organisations to their poor economic position as one income families rather than any preferential treatment given in the allocation process.

Moreover, this is not a route to housing which the young mothers in our sample who were being or had been looked after needed to follow, since care leavers were a priority group for housing under the homelessness legislation and in some local authorities their claim had also been acknowledged by housing departments under the Children Act 1989, through agreements achieved via after-care services.

The mothers and mothers-to-be in component 1 of the study recognised the prevalence of this attitude towards them but exempted themselves from such an allegation. Some were aware that they had a claim on grounds other than being pregnant. Some declared that other young women may choose this course of action but they did not. Others had simply not received any help with housing. One declared:

> 'There are a lot of things that people say about young mothers – that we have got no ambition, that we're just young people that want to get pregnant to get flats. I will tell you now, whether I got pregnant or not, I am a determined person and I would have got my own flat anyway.' (*17-year-old*)

Another young woman in a group discussion drily remarked, 'I wouldn't go through all that just to get a house.' Another, aged 16 and living in a mother and baby unit, pointed out that 'the thing about getting a house is silly because you can't even get a flat till you're 16. You have to live in a hostel till then.'

Among some young women in the care system (although not young men) there was a general level of intolerance and impatience with others who become pregnant deliberately.

> 'They just think that they know all just because they've got a baby. They couldn't have – if they had knew it all they wouldn't have got pregnant in the first place.'

> 'I've got no sympathy for people like that … Those 15-year-olds out there, they think if they have a baby everyone will admire them. I've just got no time for them.'

> 'A girl came into (the home), she was pregnant which caused major uproar cos the staff just treated her like a queen. Like, orange juice, biscuits, stuff like that all had to be bought out of our pocket money, but whenever she wanted it, she got it, they'd give it her out of petty cash, and buy things … And she was truanting, not going to school, staying in bed all day, going round her friends' houses, and staff were just letting her – they weren't doing nothing about it, and that's what caused all the

uproar cos she was just taking the mick. And then everybody else resented it cos it's not fair. I know she's pregnant and OK, so she does need a bit of special treatment to take care of the baby, but also it's a children's home – it's not equipped to look after pregnant girls ... she was having morning sickness and we had to share that bathroom and you don't want to go in when somebody's puking up, especially first thing in the morning. There's five girls all trying to get ready for school or college together, all got to be out the house, get to school on time, which they're strict on, getting out of the house, you've got to share the bathroom and she's in there for hours being sick. It wasn't fair on everyone else.'

The intolerance was occasionally tempered by an effort to understand, and, in the following case, an interview with a 16-year-old in public care by an attempt to pathologise adolescent parenthood.

'(They do it for) the attention ... when you are a mother or whatever, but to me it's stupid. There's no need to do that ... People just think that they need a baby so their life is complete but really it isn't – your life is not completed until you've lived it ... It all depends on what background you come from as well ... The thing is that they haven't got any parents or anybody to love them, so they are having a child because that child is going to love them back, give them the love and affection that they need. Them people do need help if you ask me.'
What sort of support do you think they need? (*Researcher*)
'They just need to be talked to a bit more often.'
About? (*Researcher*)
'Everything. They just need a little bit of love, but I don't see the point in having babies for love.'
Who do you think should show their love to them? (*Researcher*)
'Their mum and dad first, their parents or whoever else is there to give them the love and support.'

Such a stance contrasts strongly with that of several young women in component 2 who admitted that there had been times when they wished they had a child. One 15-year-old in this part of the study who was pregnant said that this had been her intention since the age of 12 and she had been anxious to be pregnant before her older sister. One wrote on the questionnaire 'It's a phase we go through' and another remarked:

'Some (get pregnant) because they've seen other girls older, maturer, with little babies in little Nike trainers, and little suits or whatever. That's how I was at one time. One of my friends had a baby and she was 19, and I used to think, 'I want a little baby' and that's what misleads ... cos a baby isn't a toy, it's not a teddy bear, it's not a doll.'

'Accidents' featured strongly as an explanatory factor in both samples but in the young people's terminology these encompassed both failure with contraception and failure to use it.

> 'I think 99 times out of 100 teenage pregnancies are unplanned. I don't think anyone plans a baby.' (*Male looked after*)

> 'Sometimes probably an accident, because of contraception ... Probably because they never used it anyway.'
> **Is that common?** (*Researcher*)
> 'Yes. With my friends it is, anyway!'
> **What makes them not use it?** (*Researcher*)
> 'Can't be bothered ... can't be bothered because they don't think they'll get pregnant.'
>
> (*Female looked after*)

Accidents might also include the use of drugs or alcohol:

> 'All me mates that have, like, had babies young, you know, have says, "I were pissed" or "I were stoned" or "I were fucked out of me head" or whatever they'd done. So they ended up – and half the time they just didn't bother using protection or owt like that – so they caught on.' (*Female looked after*)

> 'Depends what sort of influences they're under, like drugs, alcohol, and friends and peer pressure and stuff like that.' (*Female looked after*)

> 'Yeah, if you have a bit too much to drink you don't know what you're doing and anyone can take advantage of you, and then you get pregnant and don't know who the father is ... Like some people probably have vodka or whisky or something, so they could probably have cider or lager.' (*Female looked after*)

In one of the school groups, lack of knowledge on the part of boys was alluded to by the girls:

> 'Oh yeah, it could be an accident. Not many ... I don't know this for a fact but I don't think men and boys are very educated on contraception myself. They just mess about, don't they?' (*Mixed school group*)

However, most of the qualitative data did not support this theory. When asked whether they had any suggestions about the prevention of unplanned and unwanted teenage pregnancies our interview respondents were inclined to believe that these were not due primarily to a lack of information, but rather to the information being ignored.

> 'I don't agree one bit about the knowledge thing, because everyone is educated.

Everyone knows, even if your mum doesn't sit you down and tell you and talk about sex with you, you always pick it up off the streets.' (*Mixed school group*)

'If you give them information, probably they don't want to know.' (*Female looked after*)

'It's not just our generation. People have tried to get the message across but people aren't listening because some think, 'It's my life. I do what I want.' (*Mixed looked after group*)

'There ain't no answer, that's the honest truth.' (*Male looked after*)

Reactions to pregnancy

So why had the young women in component 1 of the study become pregnant and how had they reached the decision to carry their babies to term? As we have seen, it was not because they thought they had reached the ideal age to be a mother, which they considered to be in the early to mid twenties when there had been an opportunity to 'have lived', 'done everything you want to do', settled down, had a job and got a house. They looked largely askance at women who have children in their thirties, which they considered to be very old, but still did not believe that under 20 was appropriate, other than in certain, exceptional circumstances which they did not enjoy.

'It's all right if you're a teenager if you've got the money and the backing and the family that you need.' (*Pregnant at 16*)

One young woman stated that she had deliberately become pregnant, at the age of 15, in order to get out of the children's home where she was living. She claimed that had she been living elsewhere she would not have done so. She described herself as having been happy to be pregnant and believed that this was the method by which she could regain her mother's attention and affection, though this proved not to be the case. On a previous occasion she had tried, also unsuccessfully, to achieve the same objective by taking an overdose.

For the few with a regular partner, the pregnancy was not always unwanted; sometimes it had been planned, and their reaction to being pregnant was very positive. These women had typically been 16 or 17 at the time of conception.

However, for the majority of respondents the discovery of pregnancy was a cause of dismay and distress and remained both unplanned and, at least in its early stages, unwanted. Phoenix (1991) reported that the women in her study who were unhappy at being pregnant came mainly from the group who had considered it important not to be pregnant.

In our sample shock and disbelief were frequently the initial reactions, especially of those who had been convinced of their invincibility:

'I was numb. I just didn't feel anything. I knew I was (pregnant) but convinced myself I wasn't. I did the test and then I just sat there and cried.' (*Pregnant at 17*)

'I just didn't feel nowt. I was just numb. I didn't even think about it ... I never felt pleased. I just thought, "Oh no".' (*Pregnant at 15*)

Typically these young women had difficulty accepting and adjusting to the fact that they were pregnant. One young woman reported that it had taken her six months to make the adjustment.

The other common reaction was fear:

'When I was first pregnant I didn't want the baby and I was frightened ... I was very mixed up when I was pregnant.' (*Pregnant at 16*)

'I really was terrified when I found out I was pregnant especially the first couple of months. I really was terrified. I didn't know where to put myself, I didn't know who to tell.' (*Pregnant at 14*)

Some of the fear revolved around telling parents or carers of the pregnancy. Young mothers in one discussion group identified fear of parental/carer reaction as one of their major problems and one respondent explained:

'I think you worry more when you're living at home about getting pregnant. It's not being pregnant, it's your mum and dad, I think that's what they worry about ... I don't think it's being pregnant, it's the reaction of everyone else.' (*Pregnant at 17*)

This was the experience of one young respondent in residential care whose carers eventually turned out to be a major source of support:

'I was absolutely terrified of telling them I was pregnant, plus I was scared myself. I told D, the officer in charge, and it took me about ten minutes to tell her and she just turned round and said something like "stupid bitch".' (*Pregnant at 15*)

To our knowledge the teenagers in component 2 had not experienced pregnancy but we attempted to find out how they thought young people would react to finding themselves unexpectedly pregnant. In the series of vignettes about the relationship of a young couple (see Table A.2, Appendix B) respondents were asked to choose from a list of options how they thought the girl, Nikki, might feel on realising she was unexpectedly pregnant. By and large the findings reflected the reactions of the young mothers in component 1. Three quarters of each sample thought that Nikki would be worried about her future and about half thought she would be anxious about telling her parents or carers. However, the girls in both samples were more likely than their male peers to think she would be concerned on both these counts. A greater proportion of the boys than the girls in both samples thought that she would be happy: none of the school sample girls thought either that she would be happy or that she would be pleased because she was certain of her fertility. The looked after girls and the school sample boys were much more likely to think that knowing she was fertile would make her pleased. Both boys and girls in the looked after sample were much less likely than their peers in the school sample to think that Nikki would be worried about her boyfriend's reaction.

Abortion and adoption

Abortion is an area where the attitudes of the teenagers in the two samples of component 2 of the study differed from each other. In selecting options available to the 15-year-old who became pregnant in the vignettes referred to above, 60 per cent of the school sample compared with only 36 per cent of the looked after sample thought she might be 'wondering whether to have an abortion'. The significant difference between the samples persisted according to gender but was more especially marked in relation to the girls: 66 per cent of the school sample and 33 per cent of the looked after sample thinking that an abortion might be one of the young woman's considerations.

The same discrepancy between the samples persisted when respondents were asked to consider how the potential young father might feel. More of the looked after sample (25 per cent) than the school sample (19 per cent) thought he might be worried in case she *did* have an abortion. The differences between the samples are not significant either overall or in terms of gender but there is a greater difference between the views of girls than there is between the views of boys: those in the school sample were least likely to think this might be a concern for the young man. Conversely many more of the school sample (51 per cent) than the looked after sample (21 per cent) thought that he would be hoping that the young woman *would* have an abortion. In this case the differences between the samples were significant but especially so in the responses of boys, of whom 53 per cent in the school sample compared with only 16 per cent in the looked after sample thought that he might be hoping she would have an abortion.

There is very little research evidence on a potential father's reaction to abortion. Hudson and Ineichen (1991) claim that the general picture is that either he is not involved in the decision or that he is strongly anti-abortion.

In the discussion groups and interviews in component 2, many young people in both samples expressed a strong anti-abortion view.

'I think a lot of the reasons why teenagers have pregnancies and they don't have it aborted or anything is because they are too scared to have an abortion because they think, "Oh I don't want to kill it. I don't want to kill a kid." I know for fact if I was going to have a kid I wouldn't have an abortion ... because I'd feel like a murderer.' (*Male looked after*)

'If they just didn't think about protection or whatever, then that's their fault, but it's still not fair on the kid, they shouldn't have an abortion or anything, that's bad. Just have to do the best they can.' (*Female looked after*)

The only difference was that those in the school sample often appeared to be willing to consider abortion an option under certain circumstances (mainly connected to disability) whereas those in the looked after sample would not consider it under *any* circumstances. Even where they recognised that having the child might impose a great burden on parents, they sought alternatives to abortion.

'Like some people, like, if they have handicapped children they don't really love them and they give them away ... I'd keep it whatever it was.' (*Female looked after*)

'I think if I found out about the baby – this would be one of the hardest choices, I'd really hate this choice – because the baby was gonna come out really crippled and everything, you know what I mean, take a lot, a lot of care, like quit work, I'd really hate that. What I'd do is, if the wife didn't want it, right – not actually didn't want it, she wouldn't be able to cope with it – then I'd probably, like, get it fostered or something, get it adopted or something like that.' (*Male looked after*)

If these findings indicate stronger beliefs about abortion among young people who are looked after than among those who are not then this was strongly reflected in the qualitative interviews with mothers and mothers-to-be. Given the highly negative reactions to pregnancy it might have been assumed that abortion would be a favoured option for the pregnant young women in component 1. However, many reported a fear of telling their parents and/or carers of the pregnancy and this fear had to be faced as a preliminary to abortion. In addition, it seemed that they were subject to peer pressure not to choose a termination. A worker in an independent living unit in an inner city area commented that pregnancy amongst young women, not only those looked after, was extremely common – 'every girl between 14 and 16, if they're not pushing a pram they've got a lump' – and that other young people were extremely disapproving of those who elected to have an abortion. Moore and Rosenthal (1993) assert that teenagers and particularly 'working class girls' have the most negative attitudes towards abortion.

The sample design effectively excluded young women who had had an abortion but no subsequent or previous maternity. But as it included young mothers *or* pregnant young women it was possible, albeit unlikely, that some young women might come forward for interview who were pregnant but considering adoption or abortion. In fact none did so. However, two of the young mothers in the sample volunteered that they had had a previous termination. They had had very different reactions to the event. One had become pregnant again almost exactly one year later, an event which she described as 'spooky'. She and her partner had agreed to the abortion on practical grounds, realising that she was young (14), still at school and they had neither income nor accommodation, but this went against their emotional reactions. The other, who had been happy with the original decision, had had no further pregnancies for several years until one was planned with her then partner. These two different outcomes echo other research which points to negative outcomes if a decision to terminate a pregnancy is made in haste or under duress (Moore and Rosenthal, 1993).

The remainder of respondents were asked whether they had considered abortion as an option. The majority had not. Some stated that they did not 'hold with it' or they did not 'like things like that'. Some considered that it was tantamount to killing which they could not contemplate and many cited 'the right to live' as their reason. They were at pains to take personal responsibility for what they had done but addressed the problem in moral and emotional rather than in practical terms.

'There was no two ways about it. Abortion never came into it. And it would never have come into it at all … I just don't think it's right. I was given the right to live so I don't see why I shouldn't give the next person the right to live.' (*16-year-old with child aged three months*)

'I've never been one to agree to abortions. I just believe that everybody's got a right to live. I made the mistake so why should somebody else suffer for what I've done?' (*18-year-old with child aged two and a half years*)

'I don't believe in abortion. Because there's plenty of ways to stop getting pregnant. So I didn't think it's fair to abort a baby.' (*16-year-old with child aged two months*)

They argued that making a decision of this nature would be too difficult for them to accept throughout the remainder of their lives. These appeared not to be considered responses for the benefit of the interview but firmly held beliefs. Only one had a religious foundation: a young woman brought up in a strict faith which she had subsequently rejected nevertheless felt that she had been sufficiently 'brainwashed' in her earlier years for her to be unable to contemplate abortion.

Only two young women rejected the option of having an abortion because having the baby was a positive choice. However, their reasons for doing so were very different:

'I was speaking to my auntie at the time. I think she was, like, happy that I was still with him. And then my family found out, and other people found out and I thought, "Well it's too late to do anything". Like, people would be talking if I was to have an abortion. I did go through the stages of thinking (about it) but then I thought, "Well what have I got to lose if I keep it? There's nowt else to do".' (*17-year-old, pregnant*)

'I just said "I'm pregnant" and he (the father) wanted the baby, he was like over the moon. And I wanted the baby because the actual thought of having something that is living and being dependent on you inside you is mind-blowing and that is just a totally different experience – it is out of this world. So an abortion didn't even come into my head.' (*17-year-old with child aged seven months*)

All the young women except one had informed the father of the child about the pregnancy. Only one had suggested a termination, to which the young woman did not agree. One other, according to the young woman's account, was unhappy and confused but did not make any suggestions about what they should do. Since she was determinedly anti-abortion there was no discussion.

The remainder of the fathers were, reportedly, in favour of their keeping the baby. Again this was a purely emotional response which owed more to the 'it's my flesh and blood' school of thought than it did to pragmatic considerations. The initial reaction of the partner described as 'over the moon' was by no means uncommon, nor was it exclusive to this sample (Burghes, 1995). The one young man in the sample reported that he had told his girlfriend that if she did not want to bring up the baby he would do so although he was 17, homeless and unemployed.

The small number of young women who had decided in favour of an abortion, and who typically had already received the appointment for it, subsequently reversed their decision, feeling that they could not go through with it. This was either because they felt they could not live with the consequences or because in reality they did wish to keep the baby and had succumbed to pressure.

A social worker put forward the theory during interview that the anti-abortion stance of these young women stemmed from their feelings of rejection: they did not wish to abandon their, albeit unborn, children in the same way that their parents had abandoned them. However, it should be borne in mind that rejection by parents had not been the experience of all the young women in the sample, some of whom had done the rejecting themselves when faced with family problems. Moreover, the issue of termination was routinely addressed in wider moral terms by these young women.

The question of rejection and of its repetition arises more noticeably at a later stage when the young mothers expressed a determination that their child would not have any social worker involvement and would never enter the care system. It is also more relevant to the issue of adoption. This was a choice that was rapidly dismissed by all respondents during their pregnancy. The response of one 16-year-old, 'No, never even thought about it', was by no means untypical. Some elaborated that their own unhappy experience of living with foster carers had influenced the decision, especially when the carers had expressed an interest in adoption.

'No. I was going to be adopted and I turned round and said no ... because she used to beat me up.' (*19-year-old*)

There is little research evidence on the views of young women in the wider community about adoption although studies of pregnant teenagers indicate that, like the young women in this sample, they seldom consider it (Burghes, 1995). Anecdotal evidence suggests that, in direct contrast to the situation only some 30 years ago, pregnant young women these days are under pressure from their parents *not* to have their unplanned babies adopted.

Adoption had subsequently occurred in one case in our sample, albeit not at the young woman's instigation. Her baby entered foster care at the age of five months and was adopted at the age of one when the mother herself was still only 14.

I thought it was the best thing for her, so it weren't so hard at the time. Well it was, but it's worse now but at the time I couldn't help her or anything, she would have been better there. But you know what it's like when you're young, you don't want a baby tagging along ... Well, you believe what they tell you at the time, don't you? You think what they are telling you is right so you go by what they are saying all the time. Looking back now, I realise how silly I was to go by them, they said I can't offer her nothing but if they had left me alone and let me get on with it then things would have been different. They do pressure you a lot ... My foster parents told me I could (manage) if I was in the right place and that, but social services wouldn't help them to put me in the right place, and with support and that I could have. But I believed the social workers instead of my foster parents. (*19-year-old*)

Advice, counselling and support

From the accounts given in component 1 of the project factual information, counselling and support during the decision-making period were in very short supply. At the same time considerable pressure was allegedly put on young women to have a termination. This came predominantly from parents, carers and group workers, and, to a lesser extent, from social workers who appeared by and large not to have been involved in the decision-making process.

Young women who were living in residential care at the time they became pregnant were more likely to report considerable pressure being applied to have an abortion. It was at this stage that they felt particularly unsupported. They felt especially distressed when their problem was not addressed sympathetically and assumptions were made about their motives, as this young woman's account illustrates:

> They couldn't believe it had happened to me of all people. They thought of all people it wouldn't be me, they thought I was too wise for that to happen. But ... because I had a few friends who were going through it at the same time, one of the staff tried to make out I was copying her. Wanting it for myself, I don't know why. That was the worst thing that had happened to me while I lived there ... A lot of them said "You want to get rid of it now. You've got so many plans. Don't let this ruin it". (*17-year-old, pregnant*)

Coyne's (undated) research points to a lack of counselling available for young pregnant women: two thirds of the mothers and mothers-to-be sample (of 30) had no counselling offered. Four of the remaining ten talked to parents, of whom two advised abortion or adoption, and three to a social worker, doctor or teacher. Only two out of the entire sample felt supported and considered the help they received to be useful and unbiased.

One young woman in the sample who became pregnant at the age of 14 had sought advice and counselling from several sources although she considered only that which she had received from the Brook Advisory Centre to have been impartial. They had explained to her the implications of each of her options – fostering, adoption, abortion or keeping the baby – whereas other individuals had advised her 'Don't keep it, have an abortion, you'll regret it.' She described herself as confused and terrified but eventually decided to keep the baby.

> 'I just didn't want to have him and then give him up ... and I didn't want to have an abortion. I knew it would play on my mind for the rest of my life. I could have another baby but it wouldn't be the same baby. I really wanted to keep him ... (Abortion) was one of the options but I didn't want to get rid of him.'

However, another young woman living in the same city who also was 14 when she became pregnant reported that when she visited the Brook Advisory Centre for her pregnancy test they told her to have an abortion: 'Actually telling me, not just looking at the options, actually telling me.' She had left angrily, in haste and more determined to keep the baby.

An outstanding example of good practice was to be found in the experience of a 15-year-old living in residential care who was given both information and time to reach her own decision about the future. She did not enjoy a good relationship with her key worker and when she became pregnant and the worker was 'mentioning abortions all the time', the key worker was replaced. In a meeting with other members of staff all her options were addressed and the precise level of support that could be offered, according to what she chose to do, was set out. She was then told,

'We're not going to tell you what you can do. Once this meeting's over, it's your decision. We won't say anything else until you come to us.'

Two workers, both involved with 16–18-year-olds, were keen to allow young people freedom of choice in this area. One, working in a leaving care project stated that:

'If a young person wants to have a baby... then that's her right ... She could be a very good mother. You have to give them the opportunity to demonstrate that ... (And) because you don't feel as though you could have a termination you cannot impose that on other people.'

The other, who was working in an independent living unit where a high percentage of the young women became pregnant, was adamant that for each young woman 'it's her decision, nobody else's.' She cited the example of a colleague who could not agree with abortion on religious grounds and had therefore declined to take a pregnant resident to the hospital for her planned termination. She herself had taken the young woman, remarking that 'This is my job and it's the welfare of that young girl, not my beliefs, that counts.'

Some young women wanted their mother's help and were disappointed when it was not forthcoming, often because the mother was in favour of abortion and not prepared to look at alternatives. When asked whether anyone had been available to help them or talk to them a young couple, aged 16 and 19, described their predicament at the time:

'It would have been nice if people had been around to help us ... But no one did ... We did try a few times with my mum. But then she didn't want to know, she was just all for an abortion – "Get rid of it, go to college" and that was it.' (*Young woman*)

'My family were the same. I've got a strict family. I thought my mum would help me. She wanted to, but it was my dad. There was always trouble.' (*Partner*)

One young woman, living in a children's home, painted an even more forlorn picture of isolation:

'I phoned my mum but it was nothing to do with her because she hadn't brought me up and I phoned the baby's father and he said he would come down but he didn't ... At first I was annoyed and upset so couldn't have talked to anyone (else). Then every time I phoned my social worker she was out or busy in a meeting so I just left it.' (*Pregnant at 16*)

A total absence of pressure, information and discussion of the available options is just as likely to lead to an unfortunate outcome. This is the account of how a decision was made by a young woman and her partner who had both been 17 and living in an independent living unit.

'When O (daughter) was about a year old, me and him were going through a rough patch and we both turned round and we actually discovered that at the time neither of us wanted to keep her and we were only going along with it because we felt the other one did. Because no-one spoke to us or asked us or informed us about anything, about what was going on ... I think if somebody had spoken to us about it at the time, sat down and advised us, really told us about the future and stuff, I don't think she'd have been here now ... When I first found out I was pregnant I was really upset. I said like, "I'm pregnant" and (they said) "Oh, what are you going to do? Are you going to keep it?". "Well, I don't know." And nobody ever asked again. It was just assumed, "Well, she's going to keep it" and that was the end of it really. We just went along with everybody else ... I assumed he wanted to, he assumed I wanted to ... We was just going along with whatever anyone else wanted.'

The outcome of this, according to her after-care worker, was that the young woman realised that she had not fulfilled her potential in either education or employment and that she was very angry with her current situation:

'Frequently she says she's going to abandon the children and on one occasion ... she actually threatened to kill them.'

This is the young woman's account of what she would have liked to happen when she discovered she was pregnant.

'I don't know – get a counsellor in, just have somebody to talk to you. I mean, if you go to a clinic, an abortion clinic, they talk to you before you make a decision so, I mean, I think they should talk to you about your decision making, what it entails if you keep it and disadvantages and advantages of keeping a baby. I mean, it is hard. It would have just been nice for someone to just sit down with you both ... Because I mean, you're only kids and they're adults and they know, not us.'

This was echoed by other respondents, one of whom stated that it would have been 'useful' to have talked to someone because 'I didn't know what was happening to me'. Another, who became pregnant when she was 14, had subsequently told her social worker that if someone had told her 'how hard it is, how hard it has been, how hard it will be' then she would not have had the baby.

But not everyone would have appreciated counselling. Some felt that the decision should be made by themselves alone in their own way and in their own time. Recent research demonstrates that pregnant young women typically expect to be allowed to make such decisions alone even if this involves subsequent reliance on parental support (Tabberer and others, 1998). The young women in our sample reported feeling overwhelmed by the weight of other people's opinions, claiming that 'everyone was doing my head in' or that 'it had nothing to do with nobody else'. Others questioned the usefulness of a counsellor:

'There's no good saying, "Yeah, I'm going to see a counsellor" because it just makes you feel worse.' (*Pregnant 17-year-old*)

'Well they wanted me to see a counsellor, but I thought there's only one reason they want me to do that, so I weren't going to see one.' (*Pregnant 17-year-old*)

Making the decision about what to do was not an easy one: frequently all the available options were unappealing and a decision was made on the basis of what seemed to be the least worst option at the time. These comments came from two young women who were both 17 and pregnant:

'I only want not to be pregnant.'

'I wouldn't have been happy with any decision. It's just a shame that it happened.'

It is hardly surprising that these young women in our sample, who by and large had not been involved in decisions about their future and whose lives had seen very little long-term planning, could decide on a major issue such as this only by opting for what was least distressing to them at that particular moment. It would, in fact, be amazing if they had been able to take a long-term view when the custom and practice in their lives had revolved around lack of consultation and instant solutions to crises.

Summary points

The component 2 samples afforded some significant insights into what they considered to be the reasons for teenage pregnancies. Both samples agreed that a critical factor lay in prevention: that pregnancies resulted from young people feeling invincible or using contraception carelessly. But the looked after sample also considered that both pressure to have sex and emotional influences played a major part. In terms of pressure by boys on girls to have sex there was little difference between the samples but a significantly higher proportion of the looked after boys than the school sample boys also thought that girls put pressure on boys. However, the most significant differences between the two samples attached to emotional influences, in particular teenagers wanting something to love and girls wanting a baby, which for the looked after sample were equally important explanations for teenage pregnancies as the issues connected to prevention.

Thus, although teenagers in general may benefit from further reinforcement of messages on the need to use contraception if they do embark on sexual relationships, such messages would go only part of the way in addressing the issue for looked after young people. For them it is equally, if not more, important to help them understand and resist unwelcome pressure and to address their emotional needs. These are more serious and deep-rooted problems for which a 'quick fix' of additional basic sex education would be grossly inadequate.

The only young women in component 1 who had either become pregnant deliberately or whose baby was initially wanted were the few 'older' ones who were living with a partner. For the majority their pregnancy was a shock: they had not considered the possibility of becoming pregnant either because they were using contraception or because previous accidents had not resulted in pregnancy or simply because they suffered from the invincibility of youth. When they disclosed to the professionals involved with them that they were unintentionally pregnant they generally experienced a lack of awareness of both their current feelings and their future problems: the vast majority did not benefit from receiving unbiased information about their options or counselling to aid their decision making. They experienced considerable pressure to have an abortion, which the majority discounted on moral grounds. Because of the rejection that they themselves had suffered, these young women did not consider giving up their babies for adoption. For them, carrying the baby to term was the easiest choice to make in the short term. This is not a surprising outcome for a group of young people who are neither familiar with long-term planning nor accustomed to having control of their own lives.

The component 2 sample confirmed that, although most young people are inclined to adopt an anti-abortion stance, this is much more pronounced among young people looked after. A significantly lower proportion in the looked after sample than in the school sample thought that an option for the pregnant young woman in the vignettes might be at least to consider an abortion and the difference was especially marked in girls' responses. Similarly, when asked to consider how her partner might feel, a significantly lower proportion of the looked after sample than of the school sample thought that he might be hoping that she would have an abortion.

7 Parenthood: expectations and preparation

Since just under half of the girls under 16 and slightly less than two thirds of those under 20 who conceive continue with their pregnancy (Office for National Statistics, 1998a), attention must be focused not only on preventing unwanted pregnancy, but also on supporting those young women who choose to carry the baby to term and on preparing them for parenthood.

Local authorities have a duty to prepare young people for leaving care and the report of the Social Services Inspectorate, '... *When Leaving Home is Leaving Care ...*', emphasises that the individual needs and circumstances of young people, including those connected with pregnancy and parenthood, should be accounted for (Department of Health, 1997a). The ability to plan for cases where young women have decided to go ahead with a pregnancy was hampered by the fact that few of the authorities approached in this study had figures on the number of individuals concerned.

Preparation for parenthood had not usually been addressed at either policy or practice level. This is an area in which young people in public care might especially be in need of help and guidance if their own experience of being parented had been inadequate. These young parents might be very determined to fulfil their role successfully but may lack the knowledge and skills to do so. One large authority had recently commissioned a pack on the preparation of looked after young people for adult life of which preparation for parenthood was a part. No other authority in the study reported moving in this direction at the time of data collection for this research, although within the wider community there was a growing interest in parenting programmes.

This chapter explores teenagers' views about parenthood, both what it means to them now and how they expect to behave as parents in the future. It then looks at the experiences of the young mothers and pregnant young women in the study to see how they were prepared for their new role.

Expectations of parenthood

The teenagers in component 2 were asked on the questionnaire whether they would bring up their children in the same way as they had been brought up (Table 7.1). Not surprisingly in view of their comments in Chapter 2 more than half the looked after sample replied that they would not. A greater proportion of girls than boys thought this would be the case. Of the quarter of looked after young people who replied that they would follow their own parents' example, a lower proportion of girls than boys did so. As we noted before, girls in public care were more likely than boys to have difficult relationships with their parents and to feel unsupported by them.

In contrast the majority of the school sample thought that they would look after their children in the same way as they had been looked after. Only one fifth, significantly less than in the looked after sample, and a greater proportion of boys than girls, thought they would not bring their children up in the same way. In the school sample, respondents were more likely to reply that their children would be brought up *to some extent* as they themselves had been brought up, rather than not at all.

This was supported by the information given in interviews, where young people thought that they would emulate their parents in some respects, or would do so in spite of their intentions to do otherwise.

'My parents always looked after me, they've taught me right from wrong, so that's the way I'm going to treat my children.' (*Female school sample*)

'Probably the same as my parents. In some ways I would and some ways I wouldn't. I'd give them their own responsibility more but I'd give them some guidelines on what they can and they can't do.' (*Male school sample*)

'I suppose I'd say I'd be different but I probably wouldn't be ... I wouldn't be as stressful. They're so stressed sometimes.' (*Male school sample*)

Being understanding, along with being trustworthy and having responsibility, were the aspects of being a parent that the teenagers in component 2, regardless of whether they were in public care, identified as meaning most to them (Table 7.2). For young people living with their families the most important aspect was having responsibility, identified by 90 per cent,

Table 7.1   Will you look after your children in the same way as your parents looked after you?

	Looked after (%)			School (%)		
	Total	Male	Female	Total	Male	Female
Yes	26	34	18	46*	44	48*
No	52.5*	46*	59*	19.5	24	14
Partly	22	20	23.5	34.5*	31	38*

*Significant difference from comparative samples.

Table 7.2   **When you think about being a parent what does this mean to you?**

	Looked after (%)			School (%)		
	Total	Male	Female	Total	Male	Female
Being trustworthy	84	85	82	84	87	81
Giving praise	61*	56	65*	45	47	43
Having responsibility	88	90	86	90	87	95
Being understanding	84	79	88	77	73	81
Having the chance to do things differently if you have had a bad experience	77*	77	76.5*	56	64	46
Being strict	24	21	27.5*	22	29	13.5
Feeling tied down	31	25	37	26	27	24
Feeling proud	77	77	76.5	74	82	65
Showing and telling children you love them	91	92*	90	79	76	84
Being good fun	81*	77	84*	63	69	57
Trying to do better than your own parents did	71	60	80*	58.5	64	51
Being supportive	82	81	82	74	71	78

*Significant difference from comparative samples.

while the aspect most favoured by those in the care system (91 per cent) was showing and telling children you love them. Significantly higher proportions of those in public care than those not also rated being good fun, giving praise and having the opportunity to do things differently following their own bad experiences. Significantly more of the girls (80 per cent) than the boys (60 per cent) in public care also considered that being a parent meant trying to do better than your own parents did: the difference between the two groups of girls was also significant in this respect. This is not a surprising outcome given that many of the girls in public care in this sample had no contact or a poor relationship with one or both parents.

Although the proportions agreeing with 'feeling tied down' were similarly low in both groups (31 per cent of the looked after sample, 26 per cent of the school sample), more than a third of the looked after girls thought this was an implication of parenthood.

To try to understand more fully the young people's attitudes towards being a parent, the component 2 interviews explored what they saw as the reasons for people choosing to become parents, regardless of their age. Young people in the school sample were more inclined to regard children as an investment in the future while the looked after young people saw the instant pleasures and drawbacks.

'They want something they've created.'
'Like, complete the family. Carry on, like, your family history.'
'They want to commit to something.' (*Male school group*)

'I don't know. I mean, some people do it for the pleasure of being there for them, you know; giving them things, being able to share experiences with them. Then you get parents who have them because *their* parents want them to have them. I reckon it's just for the pure joy of having them really.' (*Female school sample*)

'The fun you can have with your kid and everything.' (*Male*)
'And you can get close with him.' (*Female*)

'And the money you get from the social, child benefit. I'm only joking!' (*Male*)
'I think it's someone that you can share your love with.' (*Male*)
'It makes you mature. Part of adulthood.' (*Male*)
'And you get more girls when you've got a kid.' (*Male*)
Does it work like that? (*Researcher*)
When you're walking round town with a baby in a pram and you get all the girls going, "Oh what a lovely baby" and then you pull the girls.' (*Male*)
What do you think are the not so good things about being a parent? (*Researcher*)
'When they start crying and they shit all over the place.' (*Male*)
'Responsibility.' (*Female*)
'It changes your life.' (*Female*)
'Your freedom. You have less freedom because you've got to look after the kid.' (Male)
'Money.' (*Female*)
'The money side, yes.' (*Male*)

(*Looked after group*)

Many of the looked after sample referred in interviews to the importance of love, sometimes in relationships with the opposite sex but more particularly as parents.

'... love's the most important but if you don't respect a child then you're not going nowhere, are you?' (*Male looked after*)

'Or even to show that baby the qualities and better – and give it a better life than what you've had, and show it a lot of love.' (*Male looked after*)

In one group discussion the young people, listing the different aspects of being a parent, quickly reached a consensus that love was the most important:

'Look, you gotta feed them, you gotta change them.'
'You gotta clothe them.'
'You gotta love them.'
'And that's the most important thing.'
'No matter what they look like.'
What do you think is the most important thing? (*Researcher*)
'Love. You gotta love your child, innit?'
'Without love it's not gonna grow up with all things it needs.'
How do you think you can show children you love them?
(*Researcher*)
'Always telling them. Holding them.'
'By you showing them, man.'
'Your body language and things. They know.'

Despite their good intentions to provide a stable and loving environment for their children and to bring them up differently from how they themselves had been brought up, looked after young people may simply not know what is involved in child care and parenting. As we have already noted in Chapter 2, their own experiences did not always offer an adequate role model. Additionally, they were much less likely than their non-looked after peers to have been given any information, either at school or in their home setting, about child care and parenthood. Looked after girls appeared to more disadvantaged than boys in learning this at school while fewer looked after boys than girls had been given information in the home setting. Significantly more boys in public care than in the comparator sample said they had been told nothing about this by parents or carers. Overall, half as many again in the looked after sample as in the school sample said they had been given no information from either source.

However, in response to a question on topics about which they wished they knew more nearly 60 per cent of the looked after sample indicated 'child care and being a parent'. As many as 70 per cent of looked after girls said they would like to know more. Although the proportions in the school sample were substantially lower than in the looked after sample, this was the topic that most young people in both samples said they would like to know more about. One young woman in a school discussion group pointed out that much more could be done about this in schools, adding, 'They tell you how to have them and how not to, but that's all!'

Joint parenting

In response to a question about whether they thought that it was better to have children within marriage, within a steady relationship, as a single parent, or whether it made no difference, neither sample in component 2 thought that having children as a single parent was a preferred option.

The looked after sample was divided almost equally among 'within marriage', 'within a steady relationship' and 'makes no difference' but boys were more inclined to choose 'within marriage' while girls tended to think that it made no difference. In the school sample, once again a higher proportion of boys than girls opted for marriage and larger percentages of girls than of boys chose 'within a steady relationship' or considered that it made no difference.

Nevertheless most respondents did not believe that parents should stay together if they do not get along. In the school sample this was particularly true of the girls who appeared to have experienced more marital breakdown among their parents than their male counterparts but who, as we have already observed, generally enjoyed positive relationships with parents' new partners. Only 49 per cent of the girls, compared with 69.5 per cent of the boys were living with both parents (with or without siblings) at the time. Twenty-three per cent, compared with 11 per cent of the boys, were living with one natural parent and a step-parent and a further 21.5 per cent, fractionally more than boys, were living with just their mother with or without siblings. In interviews the school sample girls were often vociferous on this topic, to an even greater extent than their looked after peers, despite the fact that the latter may have had more experience of their parents' marriages and relationships ending.

> 'My parents ... I don't know, they believe in you should be married before you have children, no sex before marriage and all this, you should – I don't know – just be really good when you're married, don't get divorced ... I think it's ... pretty stupid like, some of the stuff is really pathetic, like I don't agree not getting divorced or anything, because you're stuck with someone then and there's no relationship there.'
> 'Yeah, because I think it's not worth stopping with someone just because of religion, if you really hate them, it's just stupid really.'
> 'I think that's stupid as well, if you don't like somebody then you can't stay with them.'
>
> *(School sample, girls)*

The majority also agreed that 'one parent can bring up a child just as well as two parents' though in both samples many more girls than boys thought this was true and this gender difference was especially marked in the school sample. However, the qualitative data from both components indicated that most young people were not intending to be single parents themselves. Rather the majority stressed that, for the sake of the children, they would like to be in a steady relationship when they had children.

> 'A baby needs a mother *and* a father as far as I'm concerned.' (*Female looked after*)

> '... and know that there's a dad gonna be there for it. You need to have male bonding as well, don't you? Like, women can do lots of things, but

it's nice to have the dad there as well, supporting you so you don't have cope on your own.' (*Female looked after*)

'I wouldn't have children unless I had a long-term girlfriend or a wife.' **Would it matter whether you were married or not?** (*Researcher*) 'As long as I love her then it doesn't matter. Cause there's no point having a kid if you're just gonna be a one parent family ... Because it's not fair on the child.' (*Male looked after*)

'I'd do it as a couple. It'd have to be a really, really stable relationship ...' 'I mean, if the relationship's stable, the children grow up knowing the feeling of stability and hopefully they'd go into a stable relationship as well when they're older.' (*Male looked after*)

In some cases this was based on the experiences of their own parents, even where, they felt, the outcome had been successful.

'I don't wanna, like, be a single parent, because I know what it was like for my mum to be a single parent. And it were hard. So if I do have kids, even if I'm not married, I'm still going to be at home with the baby's mother.' (*Male looked after*)

'My dad left my mum before she had me and she went through it on her own, and the parents weren't very supportive and she said it was really horrible.' (*Female school sample*)

Those young women who dissented, because of their lack of trust in the opposite sex, still suggested that they would not ostracise the other parent and acknowledged the importance of a father's role in children's lives.

'Cos at the end of the day no man's gonna stick next to you ... At the end of the day if I was to have a baby, the thing would be, I'd still take the baby round to see its father, but apart from that, I think that's all.'

The vast majority of young people in both samples did not think that being a father these days was easy and boys in the looked after sample especially so. There was little difference in the level of responses from the girls (each about one quarter agreeing). Despite their acknowledgement of the difficult role for fathers, many girls in both samples had a very poor opinion of young men's attitude towards their responsibilities. Fewer than a quarter in either sample agreed with the statement that 'Young men take their responsibilities seriously': boys, unsurprisingly, were much more likely to agree with the statement with almost equal proportions (61 and 63 per cent) in both samples doing so.

In separate discussion groups with looked after children the following comments were made by young women about what they saw as the irresponsible attitude of men:

'Look at the mans of today ... if you think about it, mans don't mean it, they just breed all over, wherever they go.'

'At the end of the day, a man will have sex with you, and then the man will go away. You won't see him again, you'll be left with a baby, and no family.'

In the component 1 sample the majority of the young mothers and mothers-to-be were living alone, predominantly through choice, and they were united in saying that they would prefer not to be living with the child's father. One, comparing her experience as a lone mother with that of her coupled friends, decided that her position was preferable.

'They've got them coming in in the night time, they've got to do this for them, they've got to do that, they're moaning and if they're in a bad mood, you're in a bad mood. And I'm glad I'm on my own, me ... It would have to be what I say goes, and if they didn't like it they'd be just out of the door straight away. Because I wouldn't change my lifestyle for anyone else, no definitely not.' (*17-year-old, pregnant*)

For many, it was aspects of their boyfriend's character or behaviour which rendered him an unendearing person to have around.

'It's going to be bad enough coping with one child, never mind two!' (*17-year-old, pregnant*)

'If he offers to do anything he just does it wrong and I end up shouting. That's why I do all the cleaning myself. He offered to do it but he gets on my nerves ... I think we get on better when he's not in.' (*18-year-old with two children and pregnant*)

'I like my own space. It's nice to have a boy around, sometimes (but not to live with) – I couldn't take his smelly feet!' (*17-year-old with baby, seven months*)

'He's a real mummy's boy. Sometimes I think I'll need two prams, one for him and one for the baby ... If he thinks he's getting the mummy's boy treatment from me he's wrong. I don't do nothing for anyone.' (*18-year-old, pregnant*)

'I mean if he is here and I ask him to do something it is just as easy to do it myself than to have to sit there and nag him to do it. I would just do it myself. It used to take me half an hour to convince him to get in there and bath her. In that time I could have bathed her, bottled her and put her to bed.' (*19-year-old with child, 18 months*)

'He doesn't really respect his mum the way he should. He just slags her off and expects her to cook and clean after him and I don't want K to come home to me and disrespect me like that.' (*16-year-old with child, 16 months*)

Some had tried living with the father but this had not worked out successfully and they were happier living alone:

'Being a mother on my own was hard but then I think I've not had to put up with some moody git coming in from work and expecting his tea on the table.' (*19-year-old with child aged three years*)

'D's father was sort of there after I'd had him. He stayed around. But he weren't any help. He was more of an aggro than help.' (*17-year-old with child, 19 months*)

'I would rather be worse off (financially) and be on my own than better off and be with him. He does my head in.' (*19-year-old with child, 18 months*)

Many young women valued their own space too highly to want to share it, which may be a reaction to having spent a part of their lives either living in residential care with several other people or in foster care in someone else's home. For them a continuing relationship with distance was the preferred option.

'I wouldn't want to live together. I'd kill him! ... Because he's always under my feet and I like my own space and I can't do with anyone in my space.' (*16-year-old with baby, three months*)

'He's here all the time, but he's got his own place. I've been on my own too long, they just get on my nerves after a bit. I like to be here on my own, they get in the way, yeah ... I prefer to be on my own, because then I can get things done.' (*18-year-old, two children and pregnant*)

However, it is questionable to what extent young people on low incomes can manage to maintain separate households and financial pressure alone may be responsible for their deciding to live together. Ironically it is those who are unemployed or claiming income support who are most able to live separately when they want to as their welfare benefits are independent of each other's. A worker in a young mother's project which actively encouraged fathers to be involved with their partners and children stated that most of them still kept their own accommodation.

Some young women, despite not wanting the child's father to feature predominantly in their lives, were able to look at his role as a father separately from his role as a partner. In this respect they were not ungenerous in their assessment of his capabilities, sometimes despite evidence to the contrary.

'He's still a bit immature about it. He thinks having a baby's something that you just laugh about with your friends ... He looks after her but I don't think he realises what it is really ... He still hasn't come to terms with it. I'll just have to give him time. He could be (a good father) if he wanted to be, but he thinks more about his friends and his motorbikes and stuff like that.' (*16-year-old with baby, three months*)

'He can be (a good father) when he wants, it's when it suits him. Like the other day, he wanted to go out for a drink so he didn't want her. I said, "You can't not want her, you can have her until 8 o'clock and then go out drinking after that". But it is when it suits him. He was never bothered when we were living together. He came home from work and he would have a little play and then he would want her in bed out the way because he had been at work all day.' (*19-year-old with child, 18 months*)

In very few cases did the father offer any financial support. According to Moore and Rosenthal, (1993) teenage fathers who do not live with their partner and child are less likely to be in employment than those who cohabit. In addition, young fathers, like young mothers, usually have low levels of educational attainment and high levels of unemployment (Burghes, Clarke and Cronin, 1997). Any employment that does exist tends to be unskilled and low paid so that they are frequently not in a position to make a financial contribution. But not contributing to the cost of bringing up their child was not always the fault of the father. Some mothers did not want money if it was accompanied by the father's involvement. In addition, receiving income support was at least a more regular and reliable source of income.

While some of the fathers in this study conformed to the uncaring and indifferent feckless father stereotype, others appeared to have been pushed out of their children's lives rather than to have dropped out. Young mothers did not want them in their lives with their additional demands, smelly feet and useless offers of help. They had nothing to offer except an increased workload.

If these young men were not the ones with whom young women wanted to share their lives was that due to the fact that they were inherently unsuitable as partners? Certainly they did not, on the whole, present as a very reliable group. As we have already seen from the remarks above, mates and motorbikes still played a dominant role in their lives often to the exclusion of their family but, more seriously, a high proportion had a criminal record, a substantial number of whom had served or were serving a custodial sentence.

This was an issue that evolved in interviews rather than being addressed directly and the number identified may, therefore, not represent the whole picture. But, on the basis of proffered evidence, more than a quarter of the fathers were currently or had been in prison. Their crimes were not always stated but according to the information that was volunteered a considerable number were robbery or drugs-related offences. A relatively high proportion of young male offenders are known to be fathers and one estimate is that two thirds of those in custody are already or are about to become fathers (Pugh, De'Ath and Smith, 1994).

Their partners' imprisonment generated a mixed reaction from the young women themselves which was largely, though not exclusively, dependent on their age. Those in the younger age group (16 and under) and who had never lived with their partner tended to attempt to maintain a relationship. They took the baby with them on prison visits and tried to engage the father in their life. Some still retained hope for the future although others had had their eyes sufficiently opened for them to end the relationship.

'He's a burglar, he was in trouble with the police all the time and he goes in prison. So if he goes in prison again I'm going to tell him he's not seeing his baby. It might seem unfair but it isn't really. Because why should I let him see him?' (*16-year-old*)

'He was quite an evil man really. What I heard that he did to other people was horrible. He was locked up.' (*16-year-old*)

'I used to take her up there to see him ... I didn't think he'd be in prison for so long. Because that's one thing he really wanted, he didn't discuss it with me but I knew that he really wanted a baby ... All I think about when you say family is her and her dad really. We were supposed to be moving in together but I doubt if that'll happen now.' (*15-year-old*)

The social worker's comment on this case was that

'I think the father is still in T's life but he is, how shall I say, detained at Her Majesty's pleasure so they don't see that much of each other! T has always been very guarded with information about the boyfriend because she was worried that I was going to tell her mother.'

One young mother whose partner had said he wanted to maintain a steady relationship with her when she became pregnant was, in fact, in prison until the baby was six weeks' old. With hindsight she described this as 'a relief'. This was a more common reaction amongst those young women who were 17 or over, some of whom tended to see the imprisonment of their partner as their means of ending the relationship. There was frequently at least a hint of violence or abuse in these cases.

'He is coming out of prison after being inside for a year. That could be a big problem. He probably knows where I live and if he doesn't, his parents do. I have to move before then. Him getting in prison was the only chance for me to get away from him.' (*17-year-old*)

However, one young woman whose partner had been imprisoned presented a very different picture. She had been living with him before he was sent to prison just before the baby was born. His imprisonment had been a considerable shock to them as they had anticipated a lesser sentence.

'Oh it was horrible, it was awful. I thought he'd just get let off, that he'd be there, for the birth, there for everything. It weren't like that.'

With the help of her grandparents she made regular visits to him until his release when the baby was three months old. By this time her life had changed, she had become largely independent and this placed additional stress on the relationship which remained stormy with frequent separations. The after-care worker for both the young people (both had been looked after) had been and continued to be the main source of emotional support. She highlighted the symbiotic nature of the relationship. She thought that if it were not for W (the young woman) the father would be 'serving a very long prison sentence by now'. But W was also dependent on him:

'W is typical of many young women who have been abused in that she needs somebody with her who she feels can protect her, who she's safe with and I think she's found that in him, so ultimately he's her main source of support.'

The need for protection experienced by women who have been abused also manifested itself in the fact that several respondents currently had or previously had had partners who were many years older than themselves. One social worker referring to a young woman of 16 with a partner of 28 commented that he was 'bad news'. Another who had similar anxieties about a young woman's relationship with an older man elaborated on this:

'Well, one always has to compare what happens normally: what the normal range of things that happen in relationships is with what might be abnormal. And I would've thought that normally a 30-year-old man wouldn't be relating to a 16-year-old girl. It happens but it seems to happen in my experience when the man has an abusive character ... That rings an alarm bell.'

Early parenthood

As we have mentioned previously, many young people in component 2 had reservations about being an 'old' parent. This led a few to believe that it would, consequently, be preferable to begin having children earlier than the mid to late twenties advocated by the majority.

'It's better to be a parent if you're, like, nearer their age and then they can talk to you'
'Because you can understand what they're on about and what might be happening to them.'
'You'd get on with them better.' (*Females, school sample*)

Nevertheless there was little support for having children at a very young age. The reasons given for this covered emotional immaturity, lack of money, and not having had sufficient time or opportunity to do what they wanted to do (often leisure pursuits). In every school group having too much responsibility at too young an age was stressed and in two of these the potential for resentment, or even neglect, of the child was acknowledged.

'Not being emotionally stable.'
'At 16 you don't want to have to take a kid with you everywhere. You don't want to be looking after a kid all the time.'
'Education. You wouldn't have time for your education.'
'You wouldn't be able to hang around with all your mates and that.'
'You might neglect the kid if, like, you're young ... because you'd blame it because you couldn't go out and do the things you want to and have your education.'
'Because you don't want, like, the responsibility when you're young. And you wouldn't always know what to do.'
'When you're older you understand how to survive in life, financially, but when you're younger you don't really care.'
'You don't really know what responsibility is until later on in life and then you learn through lessons and stuff.'

(Mixed school group)

'Too much responsibility.'
'Yeah, too much responsibility, like if you were ... you'd have to grow up way before your time.'
'Say if you had a baby at 15, you'd have to act like a 24-year-old so you know what to do and that ...'
'You wouldn't be able to go out there and fulfil your dream before you settled down.'
'You've got to have a life ...'
'It all stops there, you've just got to change your life, it's a big change.'
'You've got to have a life, because if you don't have a life you just go round being depressed and you think, "I could be out with my mates now but I've got to stay in with my baby".'
'And you might might end up resenting the child in a way ...'

(Mixed school group)

Responsibility was not an issue for the looked after young people who were more inclined to stress lost opportunities, primarily those connected with pleasure, and a general closing down of life:

'The good thing is *having* a baby and the bad thing is just losing half of, most of, your life because when you're 50 and the baby's just grown up, you wouldn't be able to do anything anymore. You can't go out, like clubbing, then, can you?'

Well, some people do ... (*Researcher*)
'But they take a walking stick!' (*Male looked after*)

'Too young is 16, 19 all that business. That's too young, man, you ain't had a life.' (*Male looked after*)

'If you're 15 or something like that then your future's gone, hasn't it? Because you have to look after kids and that and you can't, like, enjoy your future and enjoy yourself whilst you're young, because you have to look after the children, don't you?' (*Female looked after*)

'Like if your friend phones to say, "You wanna go out?", you say you can't go out because you haven't got a baby-sitter or whatever.' (*Female looked after*)

'I mean, you've had no life when you're 15 and you're not gonna have no life either.' (*Female looked after*)

'If you're about 15 or something ... you can't really have a job then or anything. And then if you are living with your parents they're gonna be looking after the baby; it's gonna be more of their baby than yours.' (*Female looked after*)

Their views were not dissimilar to those obtained in component 1 where the young mothers were asked about the advantages and disadvantages of early parenthood, as well as the differences that being pregnant or a parent had made to their lives. Many of the young mothers were aware that there were no obvious advantages at this moment. They were struggling with low incomes and often with unsatisfactory accommodation. However, they could all see future benefits, which lay in two main areas. The first, and the one that most readily sprang to mind for many women, was that the small age gap would bring an increased closeness between parent and child. They believed that they would still be able to remember clearly and have empathy with the problems that beset teenagers.

'I think you'd be closer to your child.' (*16-year-old with child aged two months*)

'I think there will be (advantages) when he's older because hopefully I'm still young enough to understand.' (*18 -year-old with child aged two and a half years*)

'There's no advantages at the moment but I suppose being still young and having a teenager, because you'll be able to deal with all the problems and everything that comes up, instead of having like the 'old generation', stuck in the way you do things. Because it causes more problems, that.' (*17-year-old, pregnant*)

In addition they would be able to go out with them and enjoy shared experiences which they would not be able to do if they were older. Such experiences were very often of a precise nature:

'If you have them when you're older you can't exactly go out to a pub or club with your kid, but when you're close together you can.' (*19-year-old with two children aged two and one*)

Given that the majority of the young women themselves had young mothers and many had first been looked after during adolescence because they did not get on with their parents, it seems especially surprising that closeness and understanding are cited as the main benefit. One young woman claimed that her mother understood 'a lot more what we were going through because we were closer' although she had entered the care system at the age of 14 because of disagreements with her parents over her boyfriend.

The other main benefit quoted was that, when their children were teenagers, they themselves would still be young enough to do the things that they had been unable to do. In this sense they recognised that some aspects of their lives had merely been put on hold rather than lost for ever. Those aspects covered training, employment and pleasure.

'You can still go out and enjoy yourself when they're old enough to look after themselves. Still go out to work. If you've got no qualifications you can still train because you're young enough.' (*19-year-old with two children aged two and one*)

Some were convinced, or had convinced themselves, that the maturity and stability that they expected to have achieved by their early thirties would enable them to gain more from their deferred independence:

'When he's old enough to look after himself ... I've got my life to live then, which I think you can get more out of living your life when you're older than what you can do when you're living your life before you've settled down and everything like that.' (*18-year-old with child aged two and a half years*)

Only one mother referred to the specific pleasures associated with the child – 'loving a baby, playing with a baby, feeding a baby, caring for a baby' – while a small number felt that it forced them to alter some perceptions and increased their understanding of certain situations.

'I think you have to grow up more quickly and you know – you understand more about money and things because before I'd be at home and say, "Mum, I want this and that" and she'd say, "I can't, I haven't got enough money." I'd be saying, "Yes you have, you've got money there" but now you understand.' (*16-year-old with child aged two months*)

The other advantages that came from motherhood and that emerged during the course of interviews related to changes in character and lifestyle experienced by the young women. Some women felt that the responsibility associated with caring for a child had caused them to temper their excesses:

'And it wasn't until I actually fell pregnant with M that everything stopped and I just changed from being a little mouthy teenager to having more responsibility and accepting that.' (*19-year-old with child aged three years*)

'I think she's changed me a bit actually. Made my attitude a bit better.' (*15-year-old with child aged three months*)

'It has made me more settled in, like, myself, because I have a goal now and I have something to achieve and I have to bring her up the best way I can and give her the best of everything and do what I can to help her grow not to be like how I am.' (*17-year-old with child aged seven months*)

'Like, since I were pregnant I've really changed. I think I've changed personally ... Because I look at things different now. And I'm not always shouting like I used to be.' (*16-year-old with child aged three months*)

Others had renounced their criminal activities:

'I always used to get into trouble but now I've settled down, now I've got two kids.' (*19-year-old, pregnant and with two children aged three and two years*)

'But he's stopped me from getting into trouble with the police. He's calmed me down ... otherwise I'd probably be locked up now.' (*16-year-old with child aged two months*)

One young woman, already the mother of two and pregnant again at the age of 18, envisaged a different fate that might have befallen her:

'When I was in (the children's home) I thought, "If I don't stay out of mischief it'll get took off me anyway." If I wouldn't have been pregnant I would never have gone into the home ... I might have ended up a prostitute. You never know, do you?'

Young women were, however, also aware of the disadvantages associated with being a teenage mother. Financial hardship and loss of freedom were the two most frequently identified.

'If you can't afford to buy him clothes and things like that.' (*18-year-old with child aged six months*)

'Just the fact that you've got no money and you haven't really done much with your life and you know what you're missing and you're stuck in and everyone else is doing what they want to do.' (*17-year-old, pregnant*)

One young woman asserted that the loss of freedom was not a cause of concern to her at the age of 17 but 'if it was a person in a different position to me they wouldn't be able to cope with a child, your freedom would be more important to you than the child', although she had, earlier in the interview, referred to her initial anxieties about no longer being able to go out for a walk in the early hours of the morning if she felt like it.

Others acknowledged their lost or limited independence in a variety of ways:

'It's not easy being on your own. I suppose if you're going to have a baby at a young age, at that age there is a lot more you could be doing ... Certainly if I hadn't had her I would have thought about my career and that first.' (*19-year-old with child aged two years*)

'Like if you want to go shopping you have to get the baby dressed, everything and like ... You don't get no time for yourself really.' (*16-year-old with child aged two months*)

'You lose your freedom but you'd lose that when you get older anyway. I haven't known life without D – I was only 15 when I had him – so I can't really tell what life would be like not to have him.' (*17-year-old with child aged 18 months*)

Coping with parenthood

Young mothers tend to present late for a first antenatal appointment because they either do not realise or do not accept that they are pregnant (Simms and Smith, 1986). They subsequently attend classes to prepare them for childbirth and parenthood on an irregular basis, if at all. In our sample of young mothers and mothers-to-be only three had attended such classes; the remainder were unaware of their existence or, more typically, asserted that they 'didn't need to go'. Many of the respondents cited as their reason for not attending such classes the fact that they were already very familiar with all aspects of child care through their dealings with younger family members, often siblings from a parent's second relationship, or the children of friends. As we mentioned previously, many of the teenagers in public care in component 2 reported that they had frequently assumed a parenting role in the past.

Of the three who had attended classes two thought that they had been very instructive. The other, aged 17, who had attended a course which she described as 'a place to learn about making bottles and bathing the baby' claimed that she had learnt nothing since she knew it all from her experience with younger siblings. This view was not shared by her after-care worker who reported that the young woman had found it helpful.

One theory is that young mothers, already feeling stigmatised, consciously avoid meetings which include older mothers out of a need to protect themselves from further adverse reactions. However, this did not appear to have affected either of the two pregnant young women in our sample who had attended classes. One, aged 17, who had attended by taking an hour out of her college day reported that:

> 'I went every week. And there was a lot of people a lot older than me and they'd turn up once and you'd never see them again.'

The other, a 15-year-old who had attended with her partner, had been pleased to feel accepted into the group of older parents:

> 'It was really good. Loads of information ... Yeah, that was every week. You get relaxation, things like that. It was really good and it was nothing, a free course ... I was put on there because I was so young ... It did at first (seem strange, being young) because they sit you round. (But) nobody looked at you, stared at you or owt like that. Everybody was really pally-pally with each other.'

Two other young women had completed a child care course at school and thought that this had been helpful preparation for their own parenting but no others had received anything in terms of a programme of education for parenthood either in school or while they were being looked after. Thus, when asked how they had learned to be a parent, the reaction of one mother, aged 18, who replied, 'I didn't. It just hit me!' was not untypical. Others claimed that it had 'all come naturally' to them and they had coped well. They responded to the needs of babies with a mix of pleasure and exasperation which is common to mothers of all ages; only the extent of negative reactions may vary, given that so many of these young women had not intended to be mothers at that age. One 16-year-old mother who took delight in her baby 'when she's laughing and stuff' also referred to less joyful times:

> 'Sometimes when she screams and screams I just shout, "Get lost". It's like, just let me wake up and pretend she's not there.'

Attempts to intervene and support young women could be problematic given that, in the words of one young mother, they wanted to have a 'normal life', which she defined as 'nobody telling me what to do'. The majority were adamant that they did not want any social services involvement with their baby:

> 'And she's not going to have a social worker neither because once you get a social worker you can't get rid of them.' (*16-year-old with baby*)

> 'I don't know how well I'll look after the baby but it's not going to end up in care, that's the one thing I'm sure of.' (*18-year-old, pregnant*)

Nevertheless, good intentions are not always sufficient to see parents through, especially when they are young and alone. One residential carer who had witnessed a high proportion of care leavers becoming pregnant and lone parents commented that:

'They often say, "You won't be put in care". I hear them say that to babies and when they're about 12 months old it's, "Stop fucking crying and screaming".'

Many of the young women were in the care system because they had suffered either inadequate parenting or abandonment by parents and were therefore particularly uninitiated in what good or adequate parenting involved. An after-care worker commented that one young woman's parents were 'a right pair, that's the only way to describe them'. Some young women were deeply conscious of their own parents' failure in this area, which heightened their anxieties about their own ability to cope. And, as we saw in the component 2 sample, the majority of those who were in public care did not intend to look after their children in the same way as they had been looked after. Nevertheless the link between their past and their present in this respect did not seem to be a source of concern to many: most of those who were interviewed when pregnant stated that they thought they would make a good parent and those who were already mothers thought that they were coping well.

In most cases social workers did not raise concerns over young mothers' initial ability to manage with a baby. In interviews very few referred to a young woman's ability to parent in terms of her background and in consequence very little action was taken. This is a comment by one social worker, unusual because she had thought about the issue:

'I think I'm ashamed to say this, but the parent craft stuff you were saying about, if you look we have done absolutely nothing with the parent craft. Okay, we've been very supportive and I think I've offered – in terms of visiting and offering support and being there for court stuff – quite a good service. I've been there week in, week out, but actually sort of when (mother) begins to take over a bit of the supportive stuff, other things prioritise and you just leave it to one side. And because she's capable I've taken it for granted that she'll be okay. So I'm guilty of doing a little bit of that ... I think one of the reasons is that I thought that would be taken care of at the hospital, at antenatal ... I know they have antenatal for young women, for young parents, and I know she was interested in that but she couldn't be bothered to go. But I didn't think – I know it sounds really stupid to say – but I didn't think of looking at parent craft skills with her because I just took it for granted that (mother) would be there ... and B House (mother and baby unit) would play a role in that.' (*Social worker for young woman, pregnant when 15*)

Where anxieties on this score were voiced they emanated predominantly from after-care workers. One remarked that, in terms of her support, those young people 'who haven't experienced a great deal of family life would take priority' and another, referring to a specific case, added that 'since E has not had a good parenting experience we'd be very concerned at her ability to cope with the baby'.

One worker, describing a teenage couple with whom she was working and about whom she had some anxieties over parenting skills, commented that:

> 'I think we're too late with these two. It needed doing a lot earlier. It would be something that most young people need because nobody teaches you how to be a parent, it's really trial and error but sometimes it helps if there is somebody you can fall back on and if the extended family are not there to provide it, then you need something.'

But the young mothers themselves neither wanted nor sought help. One young woman, living alone in the community, reported that she was pleased to have been left largely to fend for herself:

> 'I might have thought they were being interfering old biddies if they had started saying "You do this". I don't know how I'd have took it . . . I didn't (learn), I just did it. It's just like with me having such a little brother – there's 11 years' difference – I've seen my mum with him. I don't know, I just did it. When I first had O me Gran came and lived with me for two weeks so she was there helping me out. I got a bit of advice from her. Other than that, I just did it meself.' (*19-year-old, pregnant at 17*)

In contrast, two mothers who had been placed for full assessment in mother and baby units, and another who had had a very brief placement in one before returning home to live with her parents, were indignant about the imposition and the implications.

> 'I said "You don't have to do anything, just leave me alone, I want to be alone with my child while I'm getting used to having a baby and have my own space and deal with it myself" . . . Basically they want to see how you are getting on with it but at that point I was really paranoid about "Why do you need to come and assess me?".' (*17-year-old, a mother at 16*)

None had been able to share the view of social workers that this could be a source of help. One 18-year-old mother who had been placed for assessment because of her relationship with the baby's father, a convicted child sex offender, said that it was 'just to see how good you were at your parenting skills. Quite awful really'. Her social worker considered that she had gained a great deal from being there and that 'her coping and caring skills' had been enhanced by her attendance.

The mothers who were living in mother and baby units were usually aware that assessment work was carried out and were keen to distance themselves from those residents who were there for that purpose:

'There's people here for different reasons, that social services are paying them to watch them, but one of them is not me ... When I first had her, everyone – they're knocking on the door, saying, "Can I do this? Can I watch you bath her? Can I do this?" But I'm thinking, "Well the hospital showed me how to bath her." I lived with my friend, my friend had a baby and I used to bath the baby and everything you know ... I refused, I said, "Don't come to my room ...". They said I haven't got a choice, but ... I said, "I don't remember ..." Even I said to my social worker, "I don't remember that I agreed to come here" and she goes, "I know, it's not an assessment home, I didn't place you in an assessment home".'
(15-year-old with baby aged three months)

Young women living in supported accommodation usually reported that they had not been given any education about parenthood while workers usually stated that it was on offer. A reason for the discrepancy may lie in the fact that young mothers moving into such places are usually asked to complete a form specifying the areas in which they would most like help so that resources can be directed appropriately. They apparently seldom indicate help with parenting skills. Another reason may be the attitude of the young women which was explained by a worker in a mother and baby unit.

'They would be asked what are their independent living skills, what would they like to learn, what do they need more practice in and what experience have they got in child care so that we can gauge whether somebody's had a bit of previous experience, perhaps from school or college or family situations, or whether somebody has got no experience or no knowledge at all. Then the key worker would give input depending on that ... There are some occasions where they (young women) seem to avoid it! The input is offered and there are hospitals that will do specific parent craft for teenage mothers and we will offer to sit down on such and such an evening and cover this topic. But some young people are quite difficult to pin down and actually commit and carry through what they said they will do.'

An additional anxiety experienced by these mothers is that they feel especially vulnerable because they are young and because they have been in the care system. They feel they are being watched and that the slightest indication of inadequate parenting will mean the social services mechanism going into operation and they could end up losing their children much more easily than other mothers who have not been looked after. In consequence their defensive attitude is not surprising.

In general teenage mothers in the youngest age groups, who are more likely to live with family or with support from others, fare better in some respects than do those who live alone in the community (Botting, Rosato and Wood, 1998). However, for those in the older age groups, living in someone else's home can be an additional source of stress (Coleman and Dennison, 1998). In our sample, those young women who lived in residential homes when pregnant or parents appeared to be more satisfied with the level and nature of help they received with parenting than those with other living arrangements. Carers often seemed to have been able to strike a balance between helping young mothers without taking over the child. This was much appreciated and even considered preferable to living in the family home with a mother who might have interfered too much.

> 'They (staff) were brilliant – always there for support. Mainly they just left me alone with J, they weren't busy-bodies.' (*19-year-old, pregnant when 16*).

> 'Like I said, without the help and support from Y House, I wouldn't have got through it at all ... I was the first one. At first I was going to have to move to a mother and baby unit, but they must've thought it wouldn't have been right for me, because I'd just really settled down there and everything. And D (manager) tried for one of the bedrooms to be made into mother and baby room, and she won that case. So I was the first one ... It were great. Because if I'd had to move into another place I don't think he'd still be here now. Because I got really close and could really trust members of staff at Y House. It wasn't like they were the carers or the workers there, they were like friends ... there's quite a few that I got that close with.' (*18-year-old, pregnant when 15*)

In one children's home the workers dealing with a very young mother particularly resistant to help found ways of dealing with this which they simply regarded as a part of their job.

> 'If B thinks you're going to lecture her then she won't listen to you, you've got to do it in a roundabout way. I mean, one of the staff bought her a load of magazines on bringing up a baby – "I don't need them". But afterwards we found her reading them. She takes advice but in her own way ... It's what it's all about really, finding out the best way to give these kids what they need.' (*Residential carer*)

Although many workers advocated the use of family centres and usually had good links with them, only one young mother had attended one. She had been just 15 at the time and living in a residential home and had been pleased to attend:.

> 'It was all right because I was just in the home all day, because I didn't go back to school ... Got me out ... They showed you how to cook and things like that. It was all right. Some of them are nosey and they interfere ... but I just told them where to shove it!'

But most young mothers are suspicious of family centres and their social services connection, fearing that to admit to needing help is the first step on the slippery road into the care system for their babies. One worker had tried unsuccessfully to persuade a young couple to attend:

'We tried to look at that (parenting) in the family centre with them once. She just wasn't interested ... The problem with family centres is they're seen as something concerning child protection issues.'

Additionally they are sometimes located in unappealing areas which do nothing to bolster the self-esteem of young mothers who are trying to prove their worth. One worker described the area in which the local family centre was situated as 'so rough even the dogs go round in pairs'.

However, despite the lack of preparation and the absence of teaching on aspects of parenting, these young mothers appeared to be faring as well as other mothers living in comparable circumstances. One social worker who was running a recently founded young parents' project in the community commented that:

'I think it was based on an assumption about young parents' abilities to actually look after children and the more I'm getting into the project and the more the assumptions are tested, these young parents are just as adequate as old parents.'

But a cause for concern is that, as one after-care worker remarked of a client, 'she prefers little babies and that's typical of most of the young women I work with'. Problems are more likely to arise when the baby becomes a demanding toddler by which time social services' involvement with the young mother may well have been withdrawn.

Summary points

Looked after young people's perceptions of being a parent differed markedly from those of the school sample in some respects: they attached far greater significance to giving praise, being good fun and having the chance to do things differently following their own bad experiences. Yet, despite their intentions to do better than their own parents had done, they were far less likely than their non-looked after peers to have been given information about child care and parenthood and the vast majority indicated this as an area about which they wished they knew more.

Though they considered that having children within a marriage or a steady relationship was preferable to having them as a lone parent – and indeed that was their own intention – nevertheless there was no agreement that parents should stay together in a state of disharmony.

Girls in both component 2 samples agreed that being a father was not easy but they also had a very poor opinion of young men's ability to take their responsibilities seriously. This was an attitude endorsed by the young mothers in component 1, many of whom had rejected the baby's father. For them, the fathers were an additional burden in their lives and provided little, if any, economic or emotional support.

There was little support from the teenagers in component 2 for having children at an early age and their reasons largely coincided with the disadvantages articulated by the young mothers in component 2: economic hardship and loss of freedom. Additionally the young people in the school sample of component 2 identified lack of emotional maturity and not having established a career while the looked after sample were more inclined to single out the loss of personal leisure time. While having children at too young an age was seen as undesirable, so, too, was having them later in life as 'old' parents were deemed to be out of touch and a source of embarrassment.

The young mothers in component 1 of the study had received little in terms of parenthood education either in pregnancy or once they became parents. They were, on the whole, unlikely to attend parentcraft classes for pregnant women. Yet their background and previous experiences of being parented suggest that they may be in need of help in establishing what is involved in good parenting. Of the professionals working with this particular group, after-care workers were the most likely to consider the abilities of young people in this area and to identify their need for help.

Once they became mothers, the main difficulty seemed to be in getting right the balance between help and interference. Young mothers both want and resist help. They have an expressed need to feel cared for, to have someone take an interest in them and their child, and yet at the same time they can, because they feel they have to prove themselves, act in a defensive manner, rejecting help that is offered on the grounds that it is tantamount to interference. A worker's definition of help may be to show young mothers the practical aspects of caring for a baby which a mother may denigrate as interference on the grounds that either she has a natural aptitude for child care or that she has had previous experience in looking after babies. The offer of help may be perceived as a checking-up exercise which will be resisted.

Some professionals were keen to engage the young mothers with family centres but these were not generally appreciated because of their association with social services and their common identification with child protection. Similarly, assessments that may be designed as much to help as to censure were not well received by young mothers who at all costs did not want to be labelled as inadequate parents. Such is their desire to prove that they have the necessary skills they will usually reject any form of guidance that is offered, no matter how informal or unthreatening it may seem to those offering it. Only those young women continuing to live with their babies in residential care appeared to appreciate the help that was offered them because this was given in a manner that was not deemed to be interference.

8   Support for young parents

The next two chapters focus on the findings relating to the young women interviewed in the first component of the study, and specifically those who were mothers at the time of interview. Attempts were made to explore the support available for these young women. Chapter 9 concentrates on the education and housing opportunities available. Here the focus is on support networks for young parents within the care system. The research also covered informal sources of support from parents, friends and partners, and these findings are outlined in an earlier report (Corlyon and McGuire, 1997).

Given that there is no comparative sample of young mothers it is difficult to assess how different the experiences of young women in or leaving the care system are from those of other young mothers, although studies such as that by Phoenix (1991) offer some insight. However, we do know that care leavers are vulnerable to economic hardship and social isolation and that many of the poor health outcomes experienced by teenage mothers are associated with a lack of economic and social support (Acheson, 1998). Consequently we might expect that young mothers leaving care fare less well than some of those living in the community and able to draw on help from friends and family.

The fact remains that the Children Act indicates that local authorities still have responsibilities towards the young parents in this study, and that their situation, however similar to that of others, must remain of concern. In summary, local authorities have certain duties and powers to prepare young people to live independently in the community, to 'advise, assist and befriend' them, to ensure that they have accommodation and, in certain circumstances, to provide them with financial assistance. However, uniform provision for care leavers is not provided throughout the country since local authorities may use their powers under the Act differently (Broad, 1994).

Transition out of care

In contrast to issues covered earlier in the report, the transition out of care and after care had routinely been addressed at policy level within the local authorities contacted. All were meeting their obligations and using their powers set out in the Children Act 1989 and had either a written procedure or policy statement on provision for young people who had been in their care and were leaving or had left.

Some of the authorities in this study had been providing programmes for transition out of care well before the implementation of the Children Act 1989 in October 1991. In one city the social services department had been offering a service to young people leaving care since 1986, initially in one district and subsequently increasing until in 1993 it provided a city-wide after-care service. With this exception the most long-standing schemes were those operated in partnership with or contracted out to a voluntary agency, either National Children's Homes (NCH) or the Children's Society. Some of these had been in operation since the mid-1980s when, as one respondent remarked, 'no-one had a clue about after care'. In contrast, several authorities had schemes that had been set up since the implementation of the Children Act 1989: one authority's policy dated from 1991, another from 1993. Yet another had an after-care project that had been operating for only 18 months at the time of the interview in August 1995.

In one authority there are four independent living units providing accommodation for 18 care leavers; two of the units can take a mother and baby placement. Referrals are made to the after-care section when a young person reaches the age of 15. The respondent's description of the process was:

> 'In real terms what that means, they're going to leave their current residential home to come into one of our resources and they're almost certainly going to get a change of social worker, because we hold case accountability in this unit, we have our own social workers here. So the young person – this was one of the criticisms we got from young people in our user survey – loses this continuity.'

The after-care team in this local authority helps young people to spend their leaving care grant and advocates on their behalf if they do not receive it. However, the amount they receive (in this authority set at a maximum of £875) is discretionary and dependent on the amount of money available in the budget. If money is not available the after-care team is powerless to provide alternative funds and can only suggest other avenues of potential support, mainly charities and charitable foundations. Pregnant young women and young mothers are usually dependent on social security money and would be directed to them for grants and loans. The after-care document on financial assistance specifically refers to money being available for child-minding facilities. This is available only under exceptional circumstances to cover periods of time in education or hospital, for example.

Bonnerjea, in her 1990 study of young people leaving care in London, found that only a small minority of London boroughs studied claimed to have or to be developing policies specifically for pregnant girls and girls with babies and that the majority of their responses were formulated in terms of practices rather than policies (Bonnerjea, 1990). In the authorities involved in our study only one had a section in the preparation and planning for after-care policy document devoted to meeting the needs of looked after young women. This states that pregnant young women have a right to all the information necessary to make an informed choice and that arrangements must be made for them to receive counselling. It also recognises the extra difficulties faced by young women who choose to have children but does not set out any provision for them. Another authority's after-care policy statement declares that 'The Department will endeavour to provide a range of accommodation which suits the needs and wishes of every young person leaving care situations, including disabled young people and those with children' – the only reference to young parents. In a third authority the policy and principles underlying the provision of after-care services state that young women have particular needs which will be met 'as a natural part of any Aftercare Service provision'. This refers to their need for a range of support and information on matters such as advice on relationships, especially sexual ones, contraception, motherhood and child care, as well as the need for suitable accommodation for young mothers. In practice they are, according to the respondent, 'persuaded to move into supported accommodation which is primarily a placement in a mother and baby unit'.

However, in at least one authority young mothers bypass the leaving care service by moving into a mother and baby unit which is expected to provide training for independence. When they move out into independent living, often as young as 16 and frequently having lost their social worker involvement, they miss out again on after-care services to which social workers might have subsequently referred them. Most hostels and homes in this sample did not offer on-going support to young mothers once they left to live in the community. This means that such young mothers are in danger of receiving less in the way of continuing support than their childless contemporaries whose passage into the after-care system has been facilitated by social workers.

Social workers

In the initial qualitative phase of the project, social workers were viewed by these young women in a very poor light, partly because of the role they had played in young people's lives in the past, which had seldom been well received, and partly due to a perceived lack of current support. There was a litany of complaints about them, in general and in particular, from young women, their partners and their parents.

Three young women enjoyed a positive relationship with their social worker. This was not necessarily based on frequency of contact. In two of the cases the young women were taken out by their social worker and indulged with time or money and in the third case the woman identified with her worker who was from the same minority ethnic group.

> 'I'm really close to my social worker . . . I do (like her), she's been with me for about nearly four years . . . I don't see her very often now because she's like doing another job . . . she works as a social worker but, like, she's took over the head social worker, so she does different things. She don't have her own cases . . . Well, she comes and sees me still. The other social worker what she give me, I didn't really like her particularly . . . (See her) probably about once a month.' (*15-year-old with baby*)

However, a young woman's view of the relationship did not always match that of her worker. One was extremely enthusiastic about her social worker and painted a picture of a close relationship in which they went shopping together and the social worker appeared to be taking on the role of an older sister. The worker had been invited to birthday celebrations and to be the godmother to the baby. The social worker's perception was that they had 'a good working relationship' but she was concerned about N's constant telephoning and over-dependence on her when she was being well supported by foster carers. She had not been impressed when N had asked to come and live with her.

In part this may reflect a young person's expectations of her social worker's role: they were frequently looking for something over and above a worker–client relationship and several of them commented bitterly that social workers saw the relationship as 'just work'.

Notwithstanding their possibly unreasonable expectations of the part that a social worker should play in their life, the young people had numerous grounds for complaint which spanned many years of social worker involvement. From the point of view of the young women, the main causes of their current dissatisfaction were that they did not listen to young people or take note of their opinions and views; they did not give honest accounts or explanations and therefore could not be trusted; they were difficult or impossible to contact; they were not supportive and did not advocate sufficiently on the young person's behalf; they were unreliable and they sat in judgment.

> 'And my social worker was useless . . . I've been without her now since November. I'm no worse off without her. I phoned her once at the office and she picked the phone up and answered it and then handed it to someone else who told me she wasn't there! But I knew it was her because she's got a Liverpool accent. She never returned the call and it was really urgent because I needed a new coat. It was the middle of winter and I hadn't got a coat. And then another time I left a message for her to ring me back and she wrote to me to tell me that she'd got the phone message but she didn't ever ring or sort out what I wanted her

to ... She should have visited regularly but it was usually about once a month. I really need someone to talk to me and listen to me as if I'm a person. After K was born I felt like she was watching me, checking up on me, asking about my feelings and how I was coping with the sleepless nights – and that was when she was three months old and I'd been coping fine.' (*16-year-old with child, aged one year*)

'They are trying to put me in a mother and baby unit, they told me that you had to stay in there for a month, "Just to look after the baby to see if you could cope and then we'll get you a flat". When we went to this meeting at the mother and baby unit it all came out, the truth: I have to stay another year and they might keep me on longer. They're saying I'm going to get grants and that, but there's a mother who's been living there for over three years. They won't let her out.' (*16-year-old, pregnant*)

One young woman had reasoned with herself that the only way forward was not to expect or rely on help:

'I think if you rely on social workers and that too much you think that they've got to do things for you ... Once you realise that they're not going to, you've just got to get on with it.' (*17-year-old, pregnant*)

When asked whether she could think of anything that would help other people avoid the experiences that she had, one young mother replied simply, 'To see the social workers more often, definitely'. She had had a particularly unhappy long-term placement with foster carers and had not been able to communicate her distress to anyone. Most of her social workers had been men. In reviews she said she would 'just sit there in the corner, going along with what they'd say because I was too scared really to speak up for myself'.

This was not an unusual case. Others claimed, for example, that in the past when they had reported abuse to their social workers they had not been believed.

'There were things going on with me and the foster father, if you understand what I mean ... I told the social worker, she didn't believe me.' (*17-year-old*)

Inaccessibility and lack of or reduced contact were particularly problematical for young women who were in a very vulnerable position. One young mother, aged 15, who spent a brief period living with her mother before taking up a placement in a mother and baby home stated:

'Well, she's only been coming to see me every two weeks since four weeks. Because before then she didn't come and see me at all. No, she only came to my mum's house to have a look at the baby and that was it. Since he was born I hadn't seen her ... She's supposed to do that anyhow from the supervision order. But she never has. And now because it's near January she thinks, "Oh, I'll come and see her every two weeks". She thinks she's smart but I'm smarter.'

The social worker's account was:

'I try to see her once a fortnight and it fluctuates between once a fortnight to once a month. I had lapsed when she was at home and having the baby, and I didn't see her for about eight weeks because I knew she was receiving really good support from mum and was at home. But I'd say over the last six weeks I've seen her once a fortnight ... she's on a criminal supervision order until January anyway as a result of the offending. And by the national standards it's supposed to be once a month. And after not seeing her for eight weeks it was like "I've missed you" and "I've been really down and I've just needed someone to talk to" and I think that made me think maybe she's not so capable ... she's not coping after all and I just felt she needed somebody outside of mum, although she was really happy with the support she was getting she just needs to have a sound off to somebody outside of the family.'

Social workers' reasons for withdrawing support were not always easy to understand. One reduced the frequent contact she had been having with the young woman because she was becoming too dependent on her. Usually they began to withdraw as soon as the young mother was seen to be coping. One social worker said that she had seen the young woman once a week when she was pregnant, reduced that to once every two weeks when the young woman went into a mother and baby home and currently was visiting about once a month 'partly because of the pressure of work and partly because she is coping well'. She would increase the contact 'if it was necessary' or if the young woman wanted her to. This is in spite of the fact that problems with children are likely to arise when they move from the baby stage and that the chances of the child becoming looked after by a local authority are greatly increased if the mother is young and single (Bebbington and Miles, 1989).

This is not an issue of individual social workers wilfully abandoning young mothers but a question of resources, as one social worker with a very troubled 15-year-old mother as a client pointed out:

'My supervisor at the moment is going "If a placement is going reasonably okay, can't you de-allocate that place?" Now to de-allocate this case would be absolute suicide.'

Some young mothers no longer had an allocated social worker and were, in many cases, relieved not to have one. But professionals who were theoretically working in partnership with local authority social workers did not share the same sense of relief. In after-care services where there was joint working with case-holding social workers, this was frequently a source of irritation to after-care workers who felt that they had, literally and metaphorically, been left holding the baby. In many cases the reason for the absence of a social worker was that one had left the team and the case had not been re-allocated, usually for economic reasons. But in other cases it was because the social worker handed the responsibility over to after care:

'There was a social worker, not a particularly active social worker. W (the young woman) was very prickly. I wouldn't like to say the word "dumped" but W was more or less put into after care and the social worker withdrew her support ... Some social workers do withdraw a lot more quickly, depending on their workload ... W has always presented as very articulate, intelligent, very capable young woman and the social worker would've had her really low on priorities, despite the fact that she was about to become a mother and the boyfriend was in prison at the time.'

Residential carers and after-care workers were very conscious of the fact that social work had become so focused on child protection that other areas of work were either passed on to other workers, such as themselves, or neglected altogether.

'With the pressures of area work, it's becoming more and more child protection focused. There is a sort of middle ground where nothing gets quite done in terms of all sorts of issues.' (*Social worker for teenage placements*)

'They expect us to feed back to them, which frees them to do more child protection work or whatever ... I think it would be nice for the young person if they did have a local authority social worker as well ... They're not always re-allocated, they're not treated as a priority, which I don't think is news to anyone.' (*After-care worker*)

A further problem in the relationship with her social worker can arise when a young woman becomes a mother and has to share any social worker support with her baby. In some cases, and especially where there are child protection issues, the baby might become the sole focus of attention to the detriment of the mother:

'What happens in the local authority is, once the baby is born then the baby's interests become paramount, which is fair enough, but what about mum?' (*After-care worker*)

Even when social workers considered that a young mother was simply another young person but with special needs they could not fail to take the child into account:

'I see S as a person in her own right but also as a young woman with a baby. The baby doesn't have her own social worker and I'm not really responsible for her but I always check on what's happening with her – to make sure she's had her injections and that the health visitor is coming regularly and things like that.'

'The roles become blurred anyway. It's really difficult, at this point because D (the baby) is doing okay, my main focus is N but you can't have N without D because you know, every time you think of N, you're going to think, "Oh she's a mother" and this brings in D. But ... I don't think there's any piece of work that should be done, whatever, to meet D's needs at this point, as far as I'm concerned. With N there's more focus, however, you've got to bear in mind that she needs time out, she needs her education, she's not just a mum.'

In one case a young mother clearly viewed the social worker as being allocated to her whereas the worker was clear that he was allocated to her child. When questioned on this he did suggest that the case might have been handled differently:

'Well, it's a question that quite honestly I didn't consider at that point in time, but in hindsight one could say that there was a child who was still ... semi-accommodated by the authority who was living with an adult sex offender, or an adult who sex offended against children, and perhaps we should have been concerned about her in her own right but as far as I was concerned the focus of our concern wasn't S, it was her unborn son.'

Some workers were clear about the need to involve another social worker specifically for the baby if there were serious concerns about his or her welfare:

'I would think, if it did come to child protection concern, they would need to be split and have two social workers, yeah. Because that's what happened on another case.'

'It's not often we would have a second worker here, not unless there were serious conflicts of interest ... There was a period before T had the baby when we were concerned we might have to remove D (the baby) ... I'd worked very hard to keep them together but I just knew I'd find it hard to separate them, and I said that if that was the course of action then I thought at that point it might be better if someone else came in and worked alongside me ... I would remain T's social worker ... I know there are occasions where you bring other social workers in to say "This is the order" and all that.'

Although there was an acceptance of the view that the baby's needs were foremost, it was not clear that this was automatically based on the legal position:

'I think there was a test case here where they were juggling with whose needs were paramount, because according to our Children Act they're both children, aren't they? And I think the court ruled in favour of the baby's needs being paramount and the child was removed.'

After-care workers

In contrast, workers belonging to after-care services were viewed in a much more positive light by young mothers and were frequently a source of support on emotional as well as practical matters. This may be due to the different roles they play in young people's lives: after-care workers who are responsible for arranging housing, organising finance, championing the cause of their clients in the face of bureaucracy can be seen to be achieving things on their behalf. Field social workers, by contrast, have never been required to make this degree of progress on practical matters. As one after-care worker explained, their role is:

'... to befriend, advise and support young people. If there's any concern regarding, I suppose, mothering, things like this, I would get a social worker.'

They do not experience the added complication discussed above of having to decide whether the needs of the young mother or those of her baby were paramount. They are always in the position of being able to see the young woman as the client even though they cannot, of necessity, divorce her needs from her role as a mother:

'My priority is with C. If I think there's any concerns between mother and baby or with L (the child) I would contact a social worker ... I chat to L, I play with L and I listen to what C's saying about him but my concerns are how C is coping in the flat, coping with L ... (But) it's not so clear cut – a lot of things overlap. Like I've taken C and L to look at schools, for milk tokens for school, for dinner tokens, so it does overlap. Because even though I'm dealing with C, L can cause problems so therefore that'll have an effect on how C is coping. So they both come, to a certain extent, together even though they are two individuals.'

However, if a serious crisis arose they would always be able to support the mother while representatives of other agencies concentrated on the welfare of the child:

'Where there is suspected child protection issues, the social worker, health visitor, whatever, will focus on the child. There is very rarely anybody offering support or advocating for the young woman and that is the role I see as the after-care worker's. Ultimately they employ social services for the safety of the baby and the child has to come first but in amongst all of that you have to be able to separate the fact that there is a young person here who probably is really hurting and needs somebody batting for their cause.'

Thus, in the eyes of young people, after-care workers could play the part of the good fairy to the social worker's wicked fairy. They help spend the leaving care grant, arrange their first independent accommodation, set them off into the world, and still have time for a cup of coffee and a chat. They do not arrange unwelcome placements at short notice or fail to provide money when it is requested. Their role is to help young people assume responsibility for themselves rather than to make decisions on their behalf.

They also have an advantage over allocated social workers in that their involvement with a young person begins on a different footing – not, usually, at a time of crisis but in a period of planning for the future. Thus the client–worker relationship can be different. This is a point made by a project worker on the advantages of after-care workers taking case responsibility. The outcome is that young people often regard them as friends rather than as superiors.

'She's all right. She came to see baby when I had baby. She's more like a friend really. She pops in now and then, sees if we're getting on all right. She's all right is T ... She helped us move and that. It were her that sorted out a grant for us moving into our first house. She gave us money for carpets and a cooker and a fridge and that, what we were entitled to, and she helped us with that ... I've got her phone number, I know where she is if I need her.' (*17-year-old with baby aged 5 months*)

One after-care worker who was working with a young woman with two children had spent a great deal of time establishing a trusting relationship with her. She felt that the young woman had been left to cope by her social worker in the mistaken belief that her claims to be managing well were the truth. Her intuition had suggested otherwise:

'We've got quite a good relationship now but it took a long time to build it up. She says herself it's only because I kept going back. I could've done what the social worker did: "This young woman looks okay, the house is beautiful, the child is beautiful, she looks all right, things look all right". But I went every fortnight and if she wasn't in I'd put a note in the door. I just kept going back because something was saying, "This isn't as good as it looks." ... So many young women like her need more and can't always ask for it.'

Some after-care workers were able to anticipate problems and make contingency plans. One had been dismayed by the lack of support offered to a 17-year-old woman being discharged from hospital with her baby at the weekend to live alone. She had made herself available:

'I didn't feel that she got the support that perhaps a young girl with a baby, knowing that she was on her own, should have got. I was a bit taken aback by the fact that they discharged a young girl knowing there's no one there to look after her . . . I nipped in for a couple of hours on the Saturday and an hour on the Sunday, just to make sure that she was all right.'

Some after-care workers appeared to be good at advocating for young people and would use creative means to achieve things on their behalf. One said that she wrote letters and 'pulled a lot of strings' when dealing with the local housing department to obtain housing for young mothers. This was always difficult if they had vacated a property that they had only recently been allocated, although she usually managed by working informally to obtain another tenancy for them. Her co-worker used the same approach:

'I'll go in there (housing department) and have a chat, a cup of coffee, just so I can push for housing for our young people! I think all contact within an agency goes on a personal level.'

Previous carers

Where the relationship with the young woman's mother was poor or non-existent, a previous foster carer often assumed the maternal role and was the person approached in a time of crisis. But not all young people were so fortunate: foster placements appeared to be either very good or very poor, and for those who had experienced the latter this avenue of support was not open. One young woman whose foster carers threw her out when she became pregnant by a member of their family found herself being physically attacked in the street by other members of this family.

Other young women retained an attachment to their residential home carers; this was a particularly marked characteristic in two of the northern authorities. Young women reported that they went back to these establishments regularly, sometimes frequently and sometimes on special occasions. They also used them as a source of help in times of crisis.

'It all depends on the situation. I turn to my mother a lot but if there's any problems I still go back to Y House, their help and support is still there. Even the members of staff, the few members of staff that started after I left and I'd not seen before, they're great. There's a bunch of members of staff that I can actually say that once you're off that list, they don't put you out altogether. I still get phone calls, he still gets Christmas presents and birthday presents, but that's out of the staff's own money. And Z who's the deputy officer in charge is great, because he just loves kids and even when he goes on holiday, M (child) gets a present, even six month afterwards, but he'll still make a point of keeping it for him.' (*18-year-old with child aged three years*)

Whether a young person's last placement had been an independent living unit or a children's home was immaterial: they maintained a strong connection with their previous carers. One residential carer thought that this was most marked with those who did not return to live with their own family but moved on to live in the community, as indeed most of the young mothers in this sample did. Much seemed to be due to the function and the attitude of the carers. Some had a remit to undertake outreach work. The carers from one residential home visited a 16-year-old mother living in the community twice a week, having offered more frequent contact which she had refused. (She reported that they 'did her head in'.) With others who were older and coping well, the position was somewhat different: there they met with young people as friends.

'It's purely friendship. I think they see us as part of their lives and, yes, I think we are important. And we certainly like to visit them ... Staff often go in their own time. And I think that's more important than going when you're on duty ... If I'm going that way I'll ring N up and say, "I'm passing through. Are you going to be in?"' (*Residential carer*)

In one case a young woman who had moved out of residential care and into her own accommodation at the age of 15, when she was already pregnant but had failed to tell anyone, was asked to come back to the residential unit in the later stages of pregnancy and when she first had the baby.

'We have had young girls with babies and they have stayed with us until they felt ready to move ... We don't chuck them out – their 18th birthday doesn't mean they've got to go ... When we heard she was pregnant we actually asked her to come back until after the baby was born ... Then we did make contingency plans and we did have staff on standby every night in case she did ring. (After the confinement) again a bed was offered to her.'

In one independent living unit, the key worker remained as the outreach worker, working alongside the after-care worker. She would visit weekly for about six weeks after a young person moved out and then fortnightly but after that 'they can always pop back and for a few months we keep them "live" ... But they know the door's always open'.

Two workers in independent living units who maintained close and caring relationships with young mothers reported that they had been told by their manager not to get so involved with current and former residents. This went against the grain of what they saw as good parenting. One described her support for a young woman, out of contact with her parents, as 'the support that a mother would give a daughter with a child'. Yet this met with disapproval:

'We've got two male supervisors and I'm constantly being told to back off a little bit ... The feelings are there but it's difficult. It will be easier when O moves from here, then I won't be being watched as much.'

Groups

The few young mothers' groups in operation were considered by users to be a valuable provision. Ironically, workers identified one of their major problems as establishing these groups and persuading young mothers to attend on a regular basis; the workers in one group organised free transport for mothers and babies to encourage attendance. Such groups, usually run by after-care services on a weekly basis; were targeted at mothers who had been in the care system and were designed to offer a forum for them to meet others in similar circumstances, to provide mutual support, to discuss problems with workers and to gain access to telephones and information. They also provided various activities which, amongst others, included art, music, first aid, understanding welfare benefits and communication skills. The mothers were involved in the planning of these programmes which were designed to offer a mix of the educational and recreational. The aim was not only to increase both the knowledge and the self-esteem of the young women but also to provide them with leisure activities that they would otherwise not be able to access.

In one young mothers' support group the workers consistently stressed the need for mothers to have time away from their babies. They had gone to considerable lengths to establish a creche facility for the one afternoon a week when they met. When the funding for this was withdrawn the workers regularly took the babies out of the room to allow the mothers uninterrupted conversations together. They strongly encouraged mothers to make arrangements for baby-sitting in the evenings so that they could engage in social activities together. They did not see this as an optional extra but as a necessity to maintain the good mental health of the young women.

Summary points

Once mothers leave to live in the community with their babies, and this can be as young as 16, they are frequently left with no support other than that which might be provided by friends or family but often is not.

Bonnerjea (1990) concluded that the ability to go back to a previous placement seemed to be the most important component of effective policies for leaving care. In this sample, in the small number of cases where maternal help was not available previous foster carers sometimes provided continuing support once young mothers left to live in the community, as did carers from residential homes and independent living units also, even in cases where after-care workers were also involved. This could continue on a long-term basis whereby the relationship evolved into friendship. However, this finding may simply be a reflection of the sample: young women who had remained in touch with residential carers were most likely to have been contacted on our behalf by those carers.

In many cases after-care workers were the only continuing support for young mothers living in the community. Like residential carers they regularly achieved a relationship with young mothers which provided both support and friendship and the young women in our sample spoke highly of their level of continuing commitment. Even if contact was infrequent and/or irregular their background presence was a source of reassurance. Young mothers leaving mother and baby units were more likely not to have engaged with an after-care service since training for independent living had, theoretically, been the domain of staff at the mother and baby unit and they therefore missed out on this valuable source of help, often leaving to live in the community without any ongoing support.

Social workers were not usually viewed in a good light by the young people, being seen more in the role of authority figures exerting control over their lives while at the same time being largely unavailable when needed. Young people often displayed unrealistic expectations about the nature of the relationship while social workers themselves frequently had to manage a demanding caseload in the face of limited resources.

A major difficulty for social workers who work with young mothers lies in establishing whether the interests of the young woman or her baby are paramount. They can easily be faced with a conflict of interests if trying to treat both equally. Once a young person is engaged with an after-care service the position becomes easier as a social worker would then become involved if necessary, should child protection issues in respect of the baby arise.

While support groups for young mothers appeared to meet with initial resistance from potential users, once established they proved to be a valuable facility, alleviating loneliness and isolation while at the same time offering leisure and educational activities.

9 Support: accommodation and education

This chapter continues with the theme of support for young parents. Crucial elements in the provision of support must be the provision of appropriate accommodation and the opportunity to continue with their education to minimise future economic disadvantage for parent and child.

Accommodation

Overview of policy and practice

Young mothers who have been looked after have been in a relatively secure position as regards accommodation since local authorities have been obliged to house them as care leavers and as a priority group under homelessness legislation. In this respect they have been in a better position than young women living with their parents when they became pregnant who, if they wished to leave the parental home to live either alone or with a partner, would usually be unable to enter their name on the local authority's housing waiting list until they reached 18 and could then often face a further two-year wait before being allocated a property (Burghes, 1995). Young people cannot hold a tenancy agreement in their own name and in some of the cases that emerged in the study tenancy rested with social services.

While not minimising the problems with entering the rented sector, the main difficulty lay in placements for young women under the age of 16.

In the interviews with the 11 local authorities, there appeared to be a lack of policies in relation to the provision of accommodation for pregnant young women and young parents. As a consequence actual provision was invariably ill defined and frequently inadequate. Again, each case appeared to be addressed separately. While the benefit of this might be that an individual's needs could be considered in the light of what was best for her, the prevailing reaction was more likely to be consternation at the absence of an accepted and acceptable route to follow and, as one respondent pointed out, the result would have 'precious little to do with what a person needs but would be bound by finance and what is there'. One female respondent described service provision in her authority for a young woman with a baby as 'lousy'. A worker in another authority wrote that in respect of policy, procedure and practice guidelines she considered that the systems in place could be discriminatory and oppressive and served only to reinforce a young woman's feelings of helplessness and lack of self-determination. She added, 'I feel these young women can be set up to fail as the hoops they have to jump through are an impossible task, and even Mother Teresa would have difficulty.'

There was, equally unsurprisingly, a variation in the provision of accommodation for pregnant young women or those with children. In one authority if a young person was 16 then the solution would be to 'move her out into the community and look to after care'. Roughly translated this meant persuading the housing department to allocate the young woman a council flat, with social services acting as rent guarantor until she reached the age of 18, and a member of the after-care team visiting her once a week. In contrast, in another authority a pregnant 16-year-old was more likely to be found a place in a mother and baby unit for a lengthy period of time. Neither of these arrangements was based on the wishes of the young woman. Other authorities were likely to 'buy into' a mother and baby unit, most of which are now to be found in the private and voluntary sectors, if there were concerns about parenting or about the baby being placed at risk.

In one city where there is a number of mother and baby units only one will accept under-16s. Social workers in the area were not always clear that a 15-year-old was eligible for a placement in this unit which meant that a valuable resource might be overlooked. However, the manager of the unit considered that it would not be a suitable placement for a 14-year-old in view of the high level of independent living. This was a view echoed by a manager in another authority who remarked that they would want to 'think long and hard about putting a 13-year-old, for example, in a 16+ unit' because of the need to support the very young mother and to recognise her developmental needs. In another authority the solution was a very radical approach which involved finding independent accommodation for the young mother, often in the community, and then providing her with 24-hour support in what was effectively her own home. The continuous support allowed her to remain in full-time education and to have the freedom to behave as a teenager. This was acknowledged to be an expensive solution but deemed, nevertheless, to be cost-effective in the long-term since it stood a high chance of allowing the young woman to be independent and in employment by the age of 18. Against this was the cost of keeping her in the care system until she was 18 and, quite possibly, the child also until the age of 18.

Regional characteristics may account for some of the variation in provision and in staff being permitted by elected members of their social services committee to devise alternative arrangements. One northern respondent claimed that, although there was no specific policy for young mothers, he thought that they did not do 'too badly' with them and in part this was due to members' attitudes which he described as 'very northern, working-class male'. By this was meant a total disapproval of young women becoming pregnant but a generous acceptance of the situation once the baby was born.

A team leader in a southern authority usefully highlighted the problems encountered by providers of services to this particular group of young women when she remarked: 'If you've been brought up in care you don't want your child to start off with any social services involvement.' She also pointed out the financial problems encountered: the budget for the provision of care services was to be cut by £300,000 in her authority which would limit even further any flexibility of arrangements for young mothers.

Foster care is an alternative which some authorities did in fact make use of, although this varied according to their level of commitment to foster care in general. In two authorities, one in the north and one in the south, it was the usual placement for pregnant girls who were beginning to be looked after. But the difficulty of recruiting foster carers willing to accept young women and their babies was recognised by several respondents. It was also an area of foster care that had not been afforded a great deal of attention, possibly because, as one respondent indicated, a priority had been given to child protection cases. Furthermore, foster carers may not exceed their approved limit so that if a young woman in their care became pregnant there might be no alternative but to find a different placement for herself and the baby.

One respondent considered that a further reason may be one of recognition. Just as authorities did not routinely collect information on young women in their care who became pregnant because to do so might constitute a recognition of a situation that needed to be addressed, so establishing a core group of foster carers specifically to cater for young parents and their children would be an acknowledgement that such provision was a constant necessity.

Information from the National Foster Care Association (personal correspondence, May 1996) indicates that of the 11,000 foster carers on their database only 11 were registered as specialising in mother and baby placements. This may not, in fact, represent the full picture since the question from which this information was culled is in an optional section of the questionnaire and was not completed in many cases. It nevertheless gives some indication of the scarcity of such placements.

Some local authorities are much more interested in using this provision than others. Again, information from the National Foster Care Association is subject to limitations but according to their available data only four authorities in England specialise in this area of provision.

Amongst the advantages of foster care for this particular group which were put forward are: it provides continuity of care which does not end when the young mother becomes independent; the placement allows for the involvement of the father in a relaxed environment without the rules and regulations attached to mother and baby units; it can offer useful male role models from within the foster family; and it can provide a model of good parenting. Its main disadvantage is one of boundaries: is the foster carer looking after the young woman or her baby or both? Is the young woman to be treated predominantly as a mother or predominantly as a young person with the needs of an ordinary teenager? Clear-cut divisions of labour and clearly defined boundaries are vital if this type of care is going to succeed. Otherwise foster carers would end up in a no-win situation where they might be accused of either not doing enough to help the young woman with the care of her baby or of taking over that care from the young woman.

Some foster placements designated as mother and baby places are for assessments, making the need for clarity between the carer and the young mother essential. In such a situation there can be no collusion between the mother and the carer: the placement has to be a clearly defined partnership between the carer and the social services department.

Residential care in children's homes is the other alternative but this raises a different set of problems related to the suitability of the accommodation and the safety of the mother and baby. Nevertheless there were some, albeit isolated, examples of good practice and imaginative solutions in this area of provision. In one authority the practice of adapting children's homes was described, which involved either basic things, such as putting in stair-gates, or making structural alterations to increase the size of a bedroom to provide a bed-sit for the young mother. Their policy was not to move a young woman simply because she was pregnant or had a baby although this would be considered if another home could provide accommodation of a more appropriate standard.

It was reported that often a very young woman who became pregnant would return to live with her family, sometimes with a parent but sometimes with a member of the extended family or with friends. It is not clear whether such arrangements were a preferred option or occurred in the absence of other provision.

Supported accommodation

The period spent in a hostel, mother and baby unit or a home is frequently seen as a necessary qualification for living independently. Consequently the time spent in this type of accommodation is seen as temporary, not freely chosen and it has to overcome considerable opposition in order to be seen as an acceptable place in which to settle. If young women experience dissatisfaction with the accommodation they are more likely to take a short-term decision to move out into what may be unsuitable housing in a disadvantaged area, necessitating a further move and more disruption in their lives. This was very apparent in group discussions where young mothers compared notes on their housing circumstances: some reported having moved out of care into properties with many problems – dampness and vermin were most frequently mentioned – which proved insurmountable. The outcome was a period of homelessness spent living with friends in overcrowded conditions while after-care workers tried to find them alternative accommodation.

Some young women appreciate having the company of others around them and this is an advantage of supported accommodation. It appeared to work well for young women when it involved living with a mixed group in terms of gender and status. The benefit was the company of other people who could spare the time to give attention to the mother and baby. Thus a young mother being accommodated in a children's home can be made to feel both cherished and important when other residents and staff want to spend time with the baby. One such woman reported that the staff coming on duty always came straight to her room to give the baby a cuddle. She appreciated this not only for the interest shown but also for the relief given to her: it gave her time to have a cup of coffee or read the newspaper for a few minutes and she particularly appreciated this if she had had a disturbed night with the baby. But she was allowed to parent the baby without undue interference from others.

Living with a group of other mothers does not offer this. Each one has her own needs and problems and has little time and energy left to show interest in another person in a similar position to herself. What could be an arena for mutual support frequently is not. On the contrary, it can become an arena for competition or withdrawal or bad feeling. One young mother who had recently left a mother and baby unit commented, 'It's all girls – it got a bit bitchy sometimes!' Another, aged 16 and still living in a similar unit, spent most of her time in her own room with her baby:

> 'I do speak to people but I'm one of these people that keeps myself to myself because I've noticed in here there's a lot of two-faced people. I don't whether it's because it's all girls but if one person walks out of the room it's "Blah, blah,blah" and then I'm thinking, "What could they say about me?" I don't really care though.'

Young people who have been looked after by a local authority frequently refer to their lack of involvement in the decisions about their life (Shaw and The Who Cares? Trust, 1998). They report that their voice goes unheard in meetings and case reviews and they are presented with arrangements that are made without their having been consulted. This is often their starting point when they move on to other accommodation, and is one reason why they are frequently so keen to obtain their own tenancy, of even the most undesirable property. If they move to accommodation that is not fully independent they do not do so in the expectation that they *will be able* to make their own decisions but rather that they *would like* to be involved in any that are made.

If, for example, they are living in hostel-style accommodation they do not appear to resent the imposition of rules and regulations as such. But they do experience problems if these are perceived to be excessive or if they do not fully understand the reasoning that lies behind them. In one mother and baby unit double futons were moved out of the residents' rooms, on the pretext that they were a fire hazard, and replaced by single beds. Residents were convinced that it was a means of discouraging boyfriends from staying, even though they were allowed to.

> 'They're a bit sneaky because – you see these futons – we used to have these in our rooms, and recently they've come out with "They're a fire hazard" so we have to have single beds put in now ... So I said I would like to buy my own double bed and they said, "No ... because it's not a double room." I said, "We had double futons. Is the reason you took the futons because you don't want boyfriends staying over?" (They said) "No. That is not the reason."' (*17-year-old*)

In another unit, bars were placed on all the windows which did not please the residents, certain that their only function was to keep out boyfriends who in this case were not allowed to stay at night. The management position was that:

> 'It was a recommendation that the health authority's inspectors required because we are in fact a registered nursing home so we have to comply with certain regulations and one of those is to make sure that the windows are safe from people falling out but in fact it has the added bonus for us of keeping the visitors out ... And I think the night staff feel quite reassured now because I think that was always quite a difficult situation when they came upon somebody in the house at night that they weren't expecting and had to ask them to leave.'

The young mothers' views were:

> 'Like the bars that have been put on the windows. They say it's for security but it's really to keep boyfriends out.' (*16-year-old*)

> 'I feel like I'm in prison. Especially the bars being on the windows ...' (*15-year-old*)

> 'I don't really like them bars because I feel – I feel inferior. Just say there was a fire and I was blocked ... I just don't feel safe.' (*16-year-old*)

Young mothers wanted their supported accommodation to be 'homely' and were disappointed when it was not. In one mother and baby unit where a unilateral decision was made by the management to close a communal room at eleven o'clock each evening the residents were extremely annoyed. One commented:

> 'This is our home at the end of the day. That's like someone coming into your house and saying that, you know "Lounge shut after eleven", then just shutting the door.' (*15-year-old*)

No matter how justifiable the reason, restrictions on the use of space, a complete ban on smoking, policies on the number of visitors allowed at any one time and set visiting times, however generous, all work against that ethos to create an environment that is more akin to an institution than a home. Similarly rooms that are decorated and equipped in an identical manner and allow little scope for individuality compound the institutional image.

In some homes and hostels there are very few restrictions on visitors and this was appreciated by residents. While it may be true that some partners present problems, others showed a considerable degree of commitment to their child by visiting on a daily basis. Such commitment might be strengthened if partners were allowed greater freedom of movement rather than being driven away. The image of the young feckless father is one that is firmly rooted in many people's minds but there may be ways in which he is helped to fulfil other people's prophecies: excluding him is one of them.

Young women's expectations of help from the staff in mother and baby units were not always met. They had been led to believe that help would be available. But the areas in which they most wanted support – practical (baby-sitting) and financial (being able to borrow money) – were not necessarily the ones that were on offer. One resident summed up the apparent feelings of many: 'To me, it always seems like they're just here to make sure your visitors go and that's it.'

Practical help

Depending on the type of accommodation, young mothers in these units often spent most of their time alone with the baby in the one room they occupied. The need for some time away from the baby can become very important to them but may be a request they find hard to formulate for fear of being considered inadequate. Some young mothers had maintained or re-formed a relationship with their own mother which incorporated some baby-sitting but others did not have this facility.

The situation is particularly difficult for mothers living communally who see other residents being able to take time away from the incessant demands of a baby. This can reinforce not only their need to have some time to themselves but also their sense of being punished and of isolation and stigma which frequently characterise their time in care. In these circumstances residents may look to staff for help, even if it had been made clear to them at the outset that such help would not be available. Such demands are not only a rational appeal for practical support but also an emotional demand for recognition. It may not be reasonable to expect staff to baby-sit: resource issues and confusion of the worker's role need to be considered. But in places where volunteer support is available this might be considered an appropriate use of their time.

Skuse (1995) argues the desirability of young mothers being able to maintain a social life. Yet in one mother and baby unit where child care was undertaken only in extenuating circumstances a worker commented that:

> 'The sort of baby-sitting that a lot of them want is in the evenings so that they can maintain their social contacts and meet up with their friends and perhaps if they were living at home there would be somebody within the family that could do that.'

Young women in the care system and for whom the state acts as a parent might have a case for arguing that the state should continue to provide the services associated with a parent when a young woman has a baby.

Financial help

Young mothers living alone are particularly prone to suffer from a shortage of money. Those who have been looked after by a local authority in residential or foster care are as unused to coping with the expenditure of day-to-day living as those who have been living with their family. It could be argued that moving into a mother and baby home at, say, the age of 15 is a useful step on the road to independent living: most bills are taken care of and the young mother receives money for her baby and herself on a weekly basis.

> 'It costs £300 to live here but I only pay £45 and 5p! I get £108 ... And then I get his child benefit soon. I think it starts on 25 December which would be £45 monthly. It's no good having it weekly, it's only £10 – that's nothing. That'd just get me a packet of nappies and some babywipes.'

But two factors are important here. Firstly, 15-year-olds do not usually have sole responsibility for feeding and clothing themselves, let alone a dependant as well. Secondly, many mothers who are older cannot manage on the small amount of money that is provided by the state. It is known (Speak and others, 1995) that debt is a severe problem for families living in the community on income support which points to the inadequacy of welfare payments. Yet looked after young mothers are usually expected to display the financial skills of an economic genius. In mother and baby units they were expected to learn how to budget so that they never ran out of money: if they did they were expected to learn a lesson from the experience and organise their accounting in a much more efficient manner in the future.

'And sometimes they have priorities for their money which is not always what staff would advise. And when you're handling your own money for the first time it's very difficult if you want to spend it in a manner that you choose ... (If their money does run out) we could put them in touch with an agency which looks at trusts and grants to see if they would be eligible in applying for certain monies but that's quite a long-winded process. So if somebody ran out of money on the Wednesday and they didn't get their next money till four or five days later, if they needed immediate support then that would be no use to them. And I think if they do get help in that sort of situation then the likelihood of them running out of money in subsequent weeks is quite high. If they run out of money and they can't go out or buy whatever it was they saw in the shops and they have to go without, then the next week, hopefully, they'll have learnt from that experience. We do allow them to make phone calls so if they want to phone their social worker or the DSS then we'd allow them to do that. And if they're out of money and it's something to do with the benefit not being correct or the giro not coming then we'd loan them the bus fare to get to the DSS but that's about the extent of it.' (*Worker in mother and baby unit*)

By contrast a worker in one leaving care unit reported that residents frequently asked him to lend them money. He agreed and was always repaid. His comment was, 'Well, that's what my parents did for me when I was 16.'

Independent accommodation

Some form of ongoing support was theoretically available to, even if it was not taken up by, all of the young women who were living in the community either alone or with a partner. Seven were in local authority accommodation, seven were renting privately and four were in housing association property. The youngest person living alone with her baby in a local authority flat was just 16 at the time of interview, although she had moved into the flat when she was 15. None of those living with partners was in a housing association property: they were most likely to be living in the privately rented sector. While not always of a standard that the young women would have liked, all of their accommodation had the advantage of not being situated in high-rise blocks of flats, even in cities where such buildings were commonplace. Of all those who were living in flats none was higher than the first floor. Moreover, none of these seemed to have suffered the extremes, identified by Speak and others in their study of young single mothers, of being offered council accommodation which is hard to let and of a highly inferior quality (Speak and others, 1995). When they had been living in sub-standard accommodation it was usually a house or flat in the privately rented sector which they had obtained for themselves. One pregnant 17-year-old found herself a house in the privately rented sector while her after-care worker was on maternity leave: she had not wanted to enlist the help of other workers because they did not understand her situation. The house turned out to be 'damp, derelict and falling apart' and strenuous efforts were being made by the after-care team to find her more suitable accommodation before the baby was born.

Most of the young women who were living independently had moved house frequently within a short period of time. One 18-year-old, already with two young children and pregnant again, reeled off a list of houses and flats she had occupied, all within the same town, in the 18 months since she had moved out of an independent living unit.

> 'I got my own house then ... off after care. And then, I went to live with F's (the oldest child's) dad. And I was there for six weeks and he threw me out and then I had nowhere to go, so I was in a refuge. And then from there I got a private house, that my mam got. Then I had loads of trouble in that street and then I moved again to the street behind, and from there I moved to here (a council house). Been all over!'

Another mother, aged 19, with a three-year-old child said that she moved out of a residential home into a two-bedroomed council flat with her baby but friends 'made a mess of it' and she had to move out. At the time of the interview she had moved into a house rented from a housing association which represented her seventh address since leaving care. Frequent changes of address are not uncommon amongst young people leaving care (Biehal and others, 1995) but nor are they uncommon in the wider community amongst the 16–20 age group. After-care workers, however, who feel they have worked hard to obtain tenancies for care leavers can often consider their efforts to have been wasted if, within a short period of time, the tenancy is relinquished. Moreover, local authority housing departments are usually unwilling to offer another tenancy, especially if the first one has been vacated in a state of disrepair or with rent outstanding.

The young women in this sample were not always successful at their first attempt at independent living. Either they found the loneliness overpowering or they had problems organising their money sufficiently well to allow them to pay bills or they allowed friends or partners to misuse their home. One young mother who, at the age of 16, moved out of a residential home where she had been very happy and into her own house found the experience quite traumatic.

> 'Towards the end you're classed as independent, which is buying your own food, paying your rent but there's nothing to prepare you for actually being around everybody to being round nobody ... Everybody gets excited about decorating and actually moving into it ... The first

night is fine, because you've got everything to do, but after that first night, then everybody just seems to have disappeared ... They (care staff from former residential home) came round to begin with, once a week, then once a fortnight ... I went down there quite a lot actually because I was that lonely. It were a good 20 minutes, half an hour walk from where I was to X House and then they turned round and said it was like me moving back in, and for my own good it would be a good idea not to come down as much ... I knew it were right. Because it was like trying to get me to be on my own, because I was down there all the time, everything was just being left.'

Because of the added responsibility of the baby there was considerable pressure for them to succeed at an earlier age than most young women who move away from the parental home. The average age for young women to leave home is about 20 (Jones, 1987) but many leave only to return again for a brief period: others at least have the option to do so. Young mothers without family support do not have this choice.

Education

One major way of countering the criticism that young mothers rely on benefit and are unable to support themselves and their babies is to equip them with knowledge and skills that will permit them to enter the job market. In practice any provision tends to be of a minimal nature. One study, concluded in 1994, indicated that pregnant schoolgirls have little chance of completing their education: although local education authorities are becoming increasingly aware of the problems, many cannot provide the support that is needed and only one third of teenagers stay on at school once they are pregnant (Dawson, 1996).

Education for pregnant schoolgirls and teenage mothers presents particular problems. Local education authorities (LEAs) have always had a power to make exceptional educational provision either at school or otherwise for pupils who have particular needs (other than special educational needs). The 1993 Education Act reinforced this provision by placing a duty on LEAs to make such provision. Circular 11/94, *Education of Pupils Educated Otherwise Than at School*, issued by the then Department for Education provided guidance on how LEAs should discharge this new duty. It advised that, where possible, pregnant schoolgirls and teenage mothers should continue their education at school; pregnancy is not, in itself, a justifiable reason for a pupil to leave school of their own volition or through exclusion. However, it is recognised that some pupils will prefer to continue their education otherwise than at school until they feel confident to return to school. Many LEAs have established pupil referral units where suitable support can be managed.

Many of the young women in this study were doubly disadvantaged, firstly by having a disrupted education because of family circumstances or by being or having been looked after, and then by being pregnant or parents. Like the young people in component 2, many had had their education disrupted by frequent episodes in the care system, by experiencing changes of placement or by entering care during adolescence. Their ability to concentrate was adversely affected by the events in their lives.

'I just couldn't concentrate: I was always on the move, in and out of care.' (*18-year-old*)

Where abuse had occurred the problems were magnified:

'I was getting all this pressure from school – "Why aren't you doing your homework?" – cramped conditions, I couldn't do anything. "Why are you not doing your homework? Why are you always late? Why is this happening? You never used to be like this, you have got potential"... It was just going on, I couldn't handle that and at home I was getting that and I was trying so hard to keep school and home away from each other.' (*17-year-old*)

When changes of placement occurred or when young people entered the care system, some local authorities attempted to maintain continuity of education:

'I went to my normal school, I kept on carrying on with the same school I went to before I left home, and I was there until I left school at 16 so it was quite good ... I think basically they left you in the school you were in and got you means of getting there which is quite good really because you don't lose all your friends.' (*19-year-old*)

In another authority this policy was sometimes pursued, even if the placement was in a different town. This usually involved providing the young woman with a travel pass but in the case of one 14-year-old special treatment was meted out and she was allowed to have a taxi to school and back. She described this as a period in which 'anything I asked for I could have'.

But others living within the same authority were not so fortunate. One young woman who had been in a long-term foster placement (11 years) was suddenly moved, requiring her to change schools, when one of her carers became ill. Despite this upheaval, and many subsequent ones, she had persevered to the extent of gaining nine GCSEs and would have continued in education had her circumstances been different:

'When I was where I was for 11 years I went to playgroup, nursery, infants, juniors. And then when I moved I did my last year at juniors and first year of high school. Then I moved to X and did the rest of high school. I were going to go to sixth form or college, because I was going to go and work at (the) racing stables, and actually got there. I was going to go and then she (foster carer) just put me out. I had nowhere to live, so I couldn't go.' (*17-year-old*)

About a third of the young women interviewed had finished their education before the minimum leaving age. Most of them had chosen to do so – one commented 'I haven't been in school since I was 14 and I just refused to do it' – but three admitted to having been expelled. In a small number of other cases their accounts of having left voluntarily did not always coincide with the explanations provided by their social workers. One who described herself as having left college voluntarily reported that she had been told she was a 'no hoper' and that her place was not in that college.

Education during pregnancy

Even if a local authority is theoretically in favour of allowing pregnant teenagers to complete their education, in practice this is by no means an easy accomplishment. Some girls leave, often despite their original intentions to remain, because of adverse reaction from their peers while others simply see it as an opportunity to abandon education which they had never enjoyed. Some schools cling on to moralistic views about the desirability of a pregnant teenager mixing with her peers and, while there is often little evidence of her being excluded specifically on moral grounds, exclusion can be achieved by citing health and safety issues (Dawson, 1996). One young woman in our study herself cited health and safety reasons:

'I was getting paranoid, because in our school on the top floor they've got these little doors and when the bell goes everybody's trying to cram through these doors, pushing through, pushing past everybody. I was getting paranoid that my baby was going to get harmed so I refused to go to school and used to go to my nan's, stay at my nan's house and then F (social worker), she referred me to this pregnancy school, so I went there to do my exams. It went all right but if I'd have just had a little bit more time in school I'd be able to show off (with good results).' (*17-year-old*)

Although social workers who were interviewed in our study were supportive of the young women being in or returning to education only one specifically mentioned it as her responsibility and stressed the future implications:

'I have a duty to see that they get some education and it's an important aspect of their life. They'll need it in the future if they want to get a job.'

One step forward is the current increase in special units for pregnant teenagers and adolescent mothers. However, their drawback lies in the inadequate provision of specialist facilities, an important issue given that the areas where these young women's education suffers most are science, information technology and modern languages.

The young women in this sample who had attended such a unit, known locally as 'the pregnancy school', had differing reactions to the provision. Some had found it a positive experience. In particular, those who had not enjoyed mainstream school and had frequently absented themselves, appreciated the shorter hours and increased individual attention that was offered.

> 'Going from full-time school to just mornings were great! And everybody that were at X matured a lot different to when I was at school ... I never did any school work until I went to X.' (*18-year-old, pregnant at 15, gained three GCSEs*)

> 'I did all the exams that I could in the time I was there but now I've missed out on the rest of the course work. They're really good there – it's supposed to be for children who are ill but you can go there if you're pregnant as well. You only go in the mornings from half past nine till half past one and there's no school uniform.' (*15-year-old, pregnant at 14*)

Another young woman had attended a special centre when pregnant at 14 but her plans to sit GCSE exams were thwarted by the premature birth of the baby. After a period of trying to manage alone and in mainstream school she eventually returned to a children's home where the staff looked after the baby and she resumed her education at the centre where she passed the exams the following year. Her social worker considered that attendance there had been the key factor in her doing so well. The unit adopted a flexible approach which allowed pupils to drop their weaker subjects and concentrate on their better ones, which greatly enhanced their chances of gaining some qualifications.

However, other young women had not been impressed by the place or by the level of education which was offered:

> 'Somebody told me I was supposed to go but then ... I was in the children's home then and I asked the person and they said no ... Well I didn't want to go schools like that because I'd been ... when I got expelled and like suspended, I used to go to them places and basically I thought they were for dunce people. They do like sums like 12 add 12 and I'm thinking, "I'm past that stage already in junior school" and I'm thinking, "Oh no." Basically I was learning things that I learned in junior school. I needed to, like, I needed for them to put me up higher but them kind of schools just give you easy work, complete easy work. That's why I didn't really want to go back. There's no point in me being at school, if there's that.' (*15-year-old, pregnant at 14*)

'I went to school till I was four months' pregnant then I went to a special school but I didn't like it there because they weren't teaching me anything even though the teachers had sent my work over. The other girls there who were pregnant didn't want to learn.' (*16-year-old, pregnant at 15*)

In this case the young woman returned to her mainstream school for the following reason.

'I was determined to go back to ordinary school because of something one of my teachers said when I was leaving to go to the special school. I said I would come back and she said "I bet you won't – they all say that and they don't come back." So I was determined to do it, just to show her. And I got seven GCSEs at grade C and she was ever so nice to me after that.'

At the time of the interview she was at college studying for 'A' levels. Family pressure and expectations, added to her determination, probably accounted for her tenacity: both elder siblings had been in higher education. A positive self-image and family background appeared to be the two main factors that distinguished those who did continue or resume their education from those who only thought or talked about doing so.

Home tuition is provided by a majority of authorities but, while Department of Education guidelines recommend 24 hours per week of lessons for 14–15-year-olds, home tuition offers them substantially less than this: the range is currently reported as between one and 15 hours a week with five hours being the most common weekly allocation (Dawson, 1996).

Some young women in the study had had the services of a home tutor but their experiences and the benefit they had obtained appeared to vary. Their perception as to whether such provision was a privilege or a penalty also varied. One young woman's mother, viewing with pride the fact that her daughter had had a home tutor and seeing it as an indication of her daughter's ability, remarked, 'You don't get them every day, do you?' The young woman, who at that time was aged 14 and had not attended school since she was 12, had appreciated the input, even though, or perhaps because, it had been minimal – about an hour a day on three days a week.

'Because when you're at school you want to do your work but it's other people about you. Because I used to do that work during the day when all the kids in the home were at school. I used to concentrate more then. At school it was the teachers that bugged me and the other kids. They always argue, don't they? ... I don't think you can concentrate. There's loads of noise and everything.'

She was less impressed by the amount of work she was asked to do, commenting, 'You should've seen the work they left you! Big pile of work!'

However, she had persevered and had passed four exams. The experience had also whetted her appetite for further education two years later:

> 'I asked D, my after-care worker. She's supposed to sort it out for me. I wanted to go to college ... I'm dead good with maths. You can get a good job when you're good with numbers, can't you? She said a woman – I don't know where she's from – she's supposed to be starting some'at up, for girls to do college work and that. They pay for child minding and stuff like that. So she's chasing it up for me.' (*18-year-old, pregnant at 14*)

Another young woman who had been pregnant for the first time at a similar age had had a home tutor but she had not continued with her work and commented that this was 'a shame really as I enjoyed going to school, I enjoyed the subjects I liked'. Her interest in further education remained diminished and although she saw herself with some form of career in the future she added, 'I don't want to have to get all those qualifications, that would do my head in.' (*19-year-old, pregnant at 13*)

However, another had had her needs met only partially by the home tutoring service:

> 'When I was pregnant and after I'd had D I had a home tutor who taught me maths but the Government wouldn't pay for another one to teach me art and that's what I was good at.' (*17-year-old, pregnant at 15*)

Young mothers and education

Completing education after the birth is no easy task but it did not defeat all the young women in this sample, although it was dependent on external circumstances as much as their own level of commitment. In one local authority two young women had widely different experiences when attempting to return to mainstream schooling after having had a home tutor. One had found considerable help and support on offer when, at the age of 14, she attempted to go back:

> 'The headmaster did say, "You can come back" and they were prepared to have someone there to look after the baby while I was at school, but then I did for a couple of days but I couldn't concentrate on my work while someone else was looking after her so I packed that in.'

The other, who became a mother at the age of 15, had found her path devastatingly blocked.

> 'I kept asking the headmaster if I could go into school to do art and he said, "Why do you want to come back now when you were always bumping off before?" Me and the tutor and the art teacher fought for me to go back at exam times because you had to have all these drawings

ready before your exams and they counted towards the exam mark. But he would only let me go in from 1 till 2, and I had to sit at the back of the class and not say anything, and from 3 till 4 when everyone had gone home. I couldn't understand it because I had never been any trouble at school.'

In our sample, one external factor which enabled young women to complete their compulsory education was the attitude of carers. Those who had been in residential care when pregnant had been supported and encouraged to continue and for those who became mothers, child care was also provided. In this way young people are both helped and hindered by being in residential care: initially it provides enhanced opportunities for both truanting and avoiding school work but subsequently it can offer a helpful environment for young mothers to achieve educationally.

Re-entry into schools is made difficult by lack of child care facilities and missed GCSE course work as well as by a dislike of formal teaching methods. Having been out of education for a long period of time compounds the problems. Further education courses, which are more likely to offer creche facilities, are one viable option for the committed. One social worker considered that a college course would suit her 15-year-old client well:

'She can't go to mainstream school because she's missed too much time and she hasn't done any preparation for GCSEs although she is bright. So it did seem the best way forward – and she said she can't cope with a school setting, that she doesn't like the teachers telling you what to do and college is better because you're more independent.'

Colleges were already being used by one or two young women and were being considered by several others. One explained the provision and her account indicated the popularity of such courses:

'I was in school odds and ends, not much. That's why they put me on to college. You can start when you're 15 but there's that many 15 and 16 years that want to go. They call it a bridge course and they pay you each week to go: to get teenagers to go. There was that many people they've had to leave it till January. They've had to try and split it up ... there's too many of us.' (*16-year-old, intending to resume education after the birth of the baby*)

However, returning to education after a long period of absence is not easy and some young women discuss this but fail to act while others embark on courses with enthusiasm only to give them up in a short period of time, unable to adjust to discipline and timetabling. Many social workers were more realistic than their clients about the difficulties attached to seeing through a course of education: one remarked of a 19-year-old with a three-year-old child who had just begun a course, 'College is early days yet, but I think if she gets to Easter she'll have cracked it.' Another, speaking of a 16-year-old with a baby, stated:

> 'I think probably she will go to college and get some sort of qualifications and go on from there, but I don't mean in the next 12 months ... She says all the right things ... We were talking about it the other day and I really believe her, it's just getting her motivated to actually go and do it.'

One young mother in the sample who went to a 16-plus college at the age of 15 having previously been out of mainstream education for two years, completed only three weeks of her course. She initially cited anxieties over child care as the main problem but subsequently claimed discrimination on the grounds of age:

> 'There were these 40-year-old teachers who'd been teaching for 20 years and they only saw me as a 15-year-old telling these people in authority what to do. If it had been a 17- or 18-year-old complaining about the college it would have been different.'

Her foster carer and social worker viewed the situation differently and felt that the young woman was by no means an innocent victim.

Three young mothers were attending college and taking higher qualifications. One was aged 16 and had a one-year-old child. She was taking 'A' levels at a college on the other side of the city from where she lived which involved two bus journeys taking an hour in total each way. She took the child with her to the creche provided by the college. During her free time, typically when everyone else did homework, she was not allowed to leave the baby in the creche with the result that she had to fit in 10 hours' homework a week.

Child care is a major problem for these young women whether they are completing their years of compulsory education or taking further education courses. The support of family and friends can make a critical difference but, ironically, many young women did not feel happy leaving their child with a grandmother because they felt that she was likely to take over the child to the detriment of the mother–child bonding process. Child care provided in creches and by child minders was, therefore, often seen as preferable; it had the additional advantage of increasing the mother's sense of independence.

A major stumbling block was the funding for this, particularly for young women over 16 who were under the auspices of a leaving or after-care programme. Several social workers referred to making application for sponsored child minding for their young clients but only one appeared to have succeeded. In fact she had succeeded exceptionally well, by achieving child minding one day a week for the young woman, aged 16 with a 16-month-old baby, not to pursue a formal educational course but to allow her time to prepare herself for entry into further education. She said that she had had to 'justify S's needs to those in higher authority' but had apparently encountered no difficulty with this.

In the same city a young woman trying to return to college to make up for lost years of education did not have a sponsored child minder and was able to take up her college place only by making her own alternative arrangements, a task that would have defeated a less determined person. In this case the social worker had not only failed to provide for her but had not informed her of his lack of success. The policy of the after-care service in this city was to provide money for child minding 'in exceptional circumstances' which were defined by the project worker as 'things like education or a spell in hospital'. But much seemed to depend on the persistence of the social worker as well as on the funds being available to meet the request.

Another, and very popular, source of education was organised by a young women's project in one town. With funding from a variety of sources, including the Workers' Educational Association, the Basic Skills Unit, Adult Education and a charitable foundation, and with a considerable amount of commitment from the project workers, they offer a range of courses covering English, maths and biology, family literacy, first aid, health issues and career advice. Many of these lead to recognised qualifications. Free child care is provided on site and this is also available to young mothers wishing to pursue educational courses provided by other institutions in the area. Young women living in a housing scheme attached to the project are also eligible to participate in the courses.

One young woman in the sample had been using the project for several years and appreciated the educational service which offered some compensation for her own disrupted school years and her eventual expulsion from school. The fact that she could gain qualifications and knowledge, obtain support and encouragement, and have some time away from the children all at the same time was very important to her.

In another town a mother and baby unit had just begun working with the basic skills unit to provide a course on family literacy for the young mothers on one afternoon a week. Reaction from the mothers in the early stages was mixed. A major drawback appeared to be that child care was not provided.

Summary points

Accommodation for all young mothers and pregnant young women without an identified home base is problematical. For many women in this sample the problems were compounded by the fact that they had not completed, and sometimes had not embarked on, training for independent living before becoming pregnant. For some the experience of being a parent for the first time coincided with a crash course in independence.

Accommodation for pregnant young women and mothers in this sample was subject to local variation. Where a mother and baby home was the usual provision, young women under 16 were particularly disadvantaged:

none would accept a referral for a 14-year-old and only one in the sample would accept a 15-year-old. Placements in mother and baby homes were not always well liked by these young women. Foster care was very limited: only one young woman was in a foster placement and several had had to leave existing foster carers when they became mothers, because either it was a short-term placement and/or it was not designated for a mother and baby. From the perspective of the young women in this sample the most satisfactory arrangement was accommodation in a children's home, or in an independent living unit if they were over 16. This offered them continuity with staff and with care but did not isolate them from their peers. It also provided them with child care if they wanted to continue in education.

A major difficulty lies in striking the correct balance between providing accommodation that both allows young mothers to be self-reliant and also offers them support and company if they either need or want it. After spending time living in the company of other young people many young mothers want complete autonomy; obtaining a tenancy of their own then assumes great importance.

Many of the young women in the study had already had their education disrupted. The provision offered in the light of their subsequent pregnancy and parental status varied greatly as did the support and encouragement they received. As a parent one of the biggest obstacles to overcome was that of finding suitable child care. All the same a number of young women in the sample had persevered with their education and many more intended to do so at some time in the future.

10 Summary and conclusions

The health and welfare of children and young people looked after by local authorities and of those leaving the care system has risen up the national and local policy agenda over recent years. In terms of the public health policy agenda, two issues are of particular concern. First, based on the available evidence, the number of young women leaving care who are pregnant or already parents is disproportionately high: indeed, the group was a focus for work within one of the Task Groups on reducing the rate of teenage conceptions and, subsequently, within the Social Exclusion Unit's remit to report on ways of reducing both unintended teenage conceptions and social exclusion for young parents. Second, in the light of the Green Paper *Our Healthier Nation* and efforts to target the neediest, this group of young mothers and their offspring are of concern to many because of the health, social and economic consequences of their early parenting. The needs of the babies themselves must be considered in their own right given the evidence on infant health and on health inequalities.

In terms of the social care policy agenda, this group of young people has already been marked out for attention. Local authorities have duties regarding sex education and responsibilities to prepare young people for adulthood as they leave care, including those young people who leave care as parents. Recent Government initiatives have reinforced the messages to local authority departments and to elected members to take better care of the children and young people whom they look after and have looked after.

With an eye to informing future interventions, this study has set out to explore why the rate of conception might be so high among young women in public care, what preparation both girls and boys looked after by local authorities receive for their role as parents in the future, and finally what support young women receive when they do become pregnant.

Summary of findings

Views and experiences of relationships

In our study many of the looked after young people had no contact with at least one parent. Relationships that did exist with parents were much worse than those experienced by their peers who were not in public care and many looked after young people reported a lack of care, attention and interest from parents. The looked after girls appeared to be particularly disadvantaged: as well as being more likely to be out of touch with their parents, they, more often than boys, reported feeling that their parents both ignored and controlled them, did not encourage them to make their own decisions and were generally less supportive of them.

Many of their parents did not act as good role models to enable the looked after young people to learn either about relationships or about parenting. Some of the parental attributes which the young people in both components reported having experienced were law breaking, alcoholism, excessive strictness, abuse, and neglect. Unsurprisingly, their view of family life incorporated violence and arguments to a far greater extent than that of their non-looked after peers.

Carers appeared to provide some compensation, especially in respect of support in school-related matters, but carers were seen to be even more controlling than parents and less likely to pay attention to young people. However, they were considered to be more helpful and caring than parents and more likely to let young people do the things they enjoyed. Nevertheless, the sum total of their carers' and parents' behaviour and attitude did not appear to match those experienced from their parents by the young people from our school sample and there was a body of looked after young people who felt ignored and controlled by both parents and carers. It is also noteworthy that in many respects boys in public care did not have such a positive attitude as girls towards their carers.

Young people in both components felt strongly about social workers' attitudes towards them. In particular they cited a disregard for their views, coupled with unreliability, unhelpfulness and unavailability as being the most distressing aspects of their dealings with social workers.

The looked after young people in our sample appeared to be given few opportunities to learn by example from the adults around them about positive relationships and in particular about trust in and from others, consideration for others' feelings and respect for their views.

Peer and sibling relationships appeared to be more satisfying to all the young people but especially to those in public care, who claimed to receive much more support from brothers and sisters than those in the comparator group who were living with their families. Looked after girls were inclined to think that their siblings trusted them and boys to think that siblings understood and listened to them to a significantly greater extent than those who were not looked after.

It was friends who generally offered most trust and understanding to all the teenagers in our sample but, like siblings, they were particularly important to the looked after group. They were also seen as the main source of respect for their ideas, a role assumed by parents in the lives of young people in our school sample. But the young mothers and pregnant young women in component 1 indicated their difficulty in maintaining friendships and their tendency to see friends as companions for leisure activities, rather than sources of emotional support.

The looked after young people in this sample appeared to rely on sexual relationships in order to feel valued and loved. Like the young people in the school sample they reported being subject to pressure from their peers and partners to have a boyfriend or girlfriend but, whereas in the school sample it was mainly the girls who reported feeling under pressure from boys, in the looked after sample boys as well as girls experienced pressure from the opposite sex. Another area of difference lay in the fact that for some looked after girls their previous experience of abuse appeared to prompt them to succumb more easily to pressure from the opposite sex.

For young people living in residential care, as most in our looked after sample were, there is additional pressure to conform to standard behaviour – in this case being in a sexual relationship – which is an important issue for a group of young people who frequently had no sense of belonging and for whom being marginalised would serve only to reinforce their feelings of rejection. Furthermore there was more scope for behaving as they wished when living in residential care where the level of individual supervision, typically associated with family life, was not possible.

Information about relationships, sex and contraception

In terms of sex education at school, there were few areas of major difference between the samples in component 2 but those that existed were important. The looked after girls were significantly less likely than those in the school sample to have been taught about emergency contraception and pregnancy while the boys had received less information than their school sample peers about pressure to have sex. This is important because, as noted above, many looked after boys considered that girls put pressure on boys and young men to form opposite-sex relationships.

Similarly, in respect of information given by carers or parents, the differences between the samples lie in crucial areas. Girls in public care were less likely than those living with their families to have been told about physical changes associated with puberty and also to have been told too late about both sexual feelings and pressure to have sex. The boys were less likely than those not in public care to have been told at all about sexual feelings, or had been told too early both about this topic and about sexual relationships. They were also more disadvantaged than the boys living with their families in learning about accessing local health services.

Many of the young mothers in the component 1 qualitative study reported having missed sex education in school and the few who had received any were critical of its timing, content and delivery. Additional or compensatory information from carers was not usually forthcoming: their input, if any, typically consisted of answering individual questions. Carers, however, are usually not trained to deliver sex education, are often unsure of parents' wishes in this respect and, importantly, at the time of interview were largely working without policy and practice guidelines in this area. If there was uncertainty among carers and social workers and a variation in their attitude towards whether, when and how young people should be given access to contraception, this is not surprising.

However, these young women were not uninformed about sex and contraception, although they appeared to have difficulty applying their knowledge. Some had omitted to use contraception at all while others claimed that it had failed. The information from the teenagers in component 2 confirmed both young people's awareness of the necessity to use contraception and their cavalier attitude towards doing so. Boys in public care were especially likely to be untroubled about a possible pregnancy and too embarrassed to discuss contraception with a new partner.

Not all the teenagers in component 2 were aware of the law in respect of sexual relationships but the looked after boys appeared more aware than any other group. On the other hand they were most inclined to think that under-age sex was acceptable, though the majority of the young people in this component, whether looked after or not, displayed a high level of acceptance of sexual activity under the age of 16.

Future expectations

In terms of education, training and employment looked after young people in the study shared many of the aspirations for the future of those who were not looked after. They also anticipated similar obstacles to obtaining employment such as lack of qualifications and training and a shortage of jobs. However, a significant difference between them was that the looked after young people also envisaged that their background and their criminal activities would be equally influential in preventing them from obtaining a job they would like and a considerable proportion of girls also believed that already having a child would do so.

For the young people in public care almost equally important as having a secure job in four years' time (when they would typically be 18 or 19) was being in a steady relationship but this was considered *more* important than having a job by the young people in the school sample. Conversely more of the looked after sample, and especially the boys, wanted both to be married or cohabiting by then and to have at least one child. This early coupledom and parenting appealed significantly less to those who were not looked after but more to boys than to girls.

Most young people did anticipate having children at some point in the future, typically within a stable relationship rather than as a lone parent. Those who were already parenting without a partner saw their future in terms of marriage or cohabitation. At the same time they looked towards having employment which would support them and their child although sometimes they had aspirations to education and employment that would be difficult to achieve.

However, looked after young people might have difficulty envisaging their future in a realistic way, if at all. The custom and practice of their lives is a series of short-term interventions at short notice in which they have no say. Unused to participating in decision making, they develop a tendency to live for the day and a fatalistic acceptance of the future.

Pregnancy

In interviews and discussions those in the component 2 sample were willing to speculate on why teenage pregnancies occur. Their reasons included a reckless approach to contraceptive use, the desire to trap a partner into a relationship and, among the looked after sample only, a means of gaining access to housing. Although some of the young mothers in component 1 also displayed a less than rigorous approach to contraception they were adamant that their pregnancies had not been planned either to keep a boyfriend or to gain a house.

From the quantitative data of component 2 it emerged that the vast majority of young people were inclined to think that teenagers became pregnant not because they did not know how to use or where to obtain contraception but because they were careless and considered themselves invincible. For the looked after boys only, an additional (and, in view of other findings, highly relevant) reason was that girls pressurise boys into having sex. But the most significant difference between the two samples lay in the equal importance which young people looked after, but not those in the school sample, attached to emotional factors, especially teenagers wanting something to love and girls wanting either a baby or to trap their boyfriends.

In the component 1 sample, the majority of pregnancies were unplanned, the exceptions being those to the few 'older' young women who were living with a partner. For the majority, general feelings of invincibility heightened by previous lucky escapes rendered their pregnancy a shock. Common reactions were fear, anxiety, dismay and distress. When they sought help from the professionals involved with them they generally met with a lack of awareness of both their current feelings and their future problems: the vast majority did not benefit from receiving unbiased information about their options or counselling to aid their decision making.

They reported considerable pressure to have an abortion, which the majority discounted on moral grounds. Because of the rejection they themselves had suffered, these young women did not consider giving up their babies for adoption. Thus carrying the baby to term was, for them, the easiest option to make in the short term. This is not a surprising outcome for a group of young people who are neither familiar with long-term planning nor accustomed to having control over their own lives.

From the component 2 samples it appeared that young people in general were predominantly opposed to abortion for moral reasons, but that those looked after were particularly prone to adopt an anti-abortion view. This was exemplified in their responses when asked to consider the possible feelings of and options open to a young couple faced with an unintended pregnancy. Significantly fewer looked after young people than those not looked after thought that neither the young woman would be considering the possibility of a termination nor the young man hoping that she would choose to have one.

None of the local authorities involved in the study had a policy framework in which to guide intervention when a pregnancy did occur even though most respondents were aware that sexual relationships of looked after young people were seen as a potentially problematical area. Pregnancies, though admitted to be far from infrequent occurrences, appeared to be addressed individually, with the professional most involved with the young woman left to deal with the situation. This was frequently unsatisfactory for the young women in question as there were clear inconsistencies in the level and quality of support that they received. However, the lack of guidance was presumably difficult for social workers and carers themselves although, because of the focus of our study, this was not explored.

Parenthood

Although half of the looked after sample had replied on the questionnaire that, four years' hence, they wanted to have had a child (which would mean before they were aged 20), in interviews they more likely to say that they did not envisage being parents at an early age, although some young women were fatalistic about the possibility of this happening. And while their desire was to have a child within marriage or a steady relationship, the girls in both the component 2 samples had a very poor opinion of young men, especially their ability to take their responsibilities seriously. This was substantiated by the experiences of the young mothers in our study, many of whom had rejected the baby's father as he was seen as imposing an extra burden on them while providing no financial or emotional support in return.

There was little support for very early parenthood for reasons that were similar to those articulated by the component 1 mothers – predominantly lack of money and loss of freedom. However, those young women interviewed who were already mothers or mothers-to-be found some benefits in their situation, the main one being the way in which their behaviour had changed: many considered themselves to have become more responsible and less prone to deviancy as a consequence of motherhood.

For the future they felt that the small age gap between themselves and their children would afford them extra understanding of their child, apparently unaware that this had not necessarily been their own experience of having a young mother. For very many of the young people in our study having children late in life was seen as inadvisable as having them early as old parents were perceived to be lacking understanding and a potential source of embarrassment to their children.

The majority of the looked after young people in component 2 saw parenthood as an opportunity to compensate for their own adverse experiences of being parented. This was not a view shared by the teenagers in the school sample who also, as potential parents, attached much less significance than those in public care to giving praise, showing affection and sharing enjoyment with a child. While the looked after group did not intend, on the whole, to bring up their children in the same way as they had been brought up, they had been provided with very little information, and certainly less than their non-looked after peers, about family life and child care. Many expressed a desire for more information on these topics.

The young mothers in component 2 had received little in terms of parenthood education either in pregnancy or once they became parents and they were unlikely to have attended parentcraft classes for pregnant women. This reluctance to access services or perhaps ignorance of services is a matter of concern since studies have shown that good antenatal care is associated with improved pregnancy outcomes for teenagers as well as older women. In addition, infant mortality is highest for the under twenties, and health patterns for childhood and for life thereafter can be affected before birth.

The background and previous experiences of many suggested a need for help in establishing patterns of good parenting. Of the professionals working with this particular group, after-care workers were the most likely to consider the abilities of young people in this area and to identify their need for help. Many mothers have difficulty asking for help with what is, theoretically, a natural process but for those who are young and have been in public care the difficulty is compounded. While they want help they will also resist it, feeling they have to prove themselves. A worker's attempt to show the practical aspects of caring for a baby may be denigrated by a young mother on the grounds that she has a natural aptitude for child care or that she has had previous experience in looking after babies. The offer of help may be perceived as tantamount to interference or, even worse, as a checking-up exercise to be avoided at all costs because of its implications.

Some professionals were keen to engage the young mothers with family centres but their association with social services and their common identification with child protection posed an even greater threat to mothers already feeling vulnerable. Similarly, assessments, which may be designed as much to help as to censure, were not well received. Only those young women continuing to live with their babies in residential care appeared to appreciate the help that was offered them because this was given in a manner deemed to be neither threatening nor interfering.

Support in parenthood

The literature suggests that the consequences of teenage pregnancy need not be adverse if the mother has a supportive network. Once the mothers in our sample left to live in the community with their babies, and this could be as young as 16, they were sometimes left with no support other than that which might be provided by friends or family but often was not.

Many experienced difficulty in either building or maintaining relationships and accepting support. Some were ambivalent about the role they wished the baby's father to play in their lives. In some cases the arrival of a baby heralded the renewal of a relationship between the young woman and her own mother, though this often raised concerns among the professionals involved in view of the mother's own proven lack of parenting skills. It also meant that some young mothers simply gave support to their mothers without receiving any in return.

Where maternal help was not available, previous foster carers and carers from residential homes and independent living units sometimes provided continuing support, alongside or instead of after-care service provision. This typically continued on a long-term basis, evolving into friendship. However, this finding may be a reflection of the sample since residential carers were most likely to have contacted on our behalf those young women with whom they had remained in touch.

In many cases after-care workers were the only continuing support for young mothers living in the community. Like residential carers they regularly achieved a relationship with young mothers which provided both support and friendship and the young women in our sample spoke highly of their level of continuing commitment, even when contact was infrequent and/or irregular. Young mothers leaving mother and baby units were most likely to be at a disadvantage in this respect. Since training for independent living had, theoretically, been the domain of staff at the mother and baby unit they seldom engaged with an after-care service and were likely to live in the community without any ongoing support.

The young mothers continued to view social workers in a poor light, invariably owing to what they saw as a previous negligent, indifferent but controlling attitude towards them. Some young people, however, entertained unrealistic expectations about the nature of the relationship, while the volume and nature of social workers' work meant they could not give priority to the young mothers. A major difficulty for social workers working with young mothers was in establishing whether the interests of the young woman or the baby were paramount and this appeared to be an unresolved issue for many. Once a young person is engaged with an after-care service the position becomes easier as a social worker would become involved if child protection issues in respect of the baby arose, leaving the after-care worker to continue supporting the mother.

While support groups for young mothers appeared to meet with initial resistance from potential users, once established they proved to be a valuable facility, alleviating loneliness and isolation while at the same time offering leisure and educational activities.

Many of the younger women in this sample had not completed, and some had not even begun, training for independent living before becoming pregnant. This compounded the problems of finding suitable accommodation for them. In fact, appropriate supported accommodation for the mothers and expectant mothers in this sample was subject to local variation but in general young women under 16 were particularly disadvantaged. No mother and baby home in our sample would accept a 14-year-old and only one would accept a 15-year-old. These placements were seldom liked by young mothers. Foster care, which might have been a more popular option, was very limited and only one young woman in our sample was in a foster placement. Once they had had the baby some had had to leave existing foster carers for bureaucratic rather than personal reasons. Those who remained in a children's home, or in an independent living unit if they were over 16, appeared to fare best as these afforded continuity with staff, with care and with their peers. In exceptional cases they might also provide child care to allow a young mother to continue in education.

In common with those leaving care without children, many young mothers want complete autonomy over their living arrangements and having their own accommodation is of great importance. However, some still desire the company of others and a difficulty for service providers lies in providing accommodation that both allows young mothers to be independent but does not exclude or isolate. It was rare in our sample to find supported accommodation which encouraged fathers to be involved with their partner and child, and this served only to drive fathers further out of the picture.

Many of the young women in the study had already had their education disrupted or terminated. The provision, support and encouragement they received once pregnant or parents varied greatly. A major obstacle to resuming education after the birth was finding and funding child care. Nevertheless a small number of young women in the sample had persevered with their education and many more expressed an intention to do so.

Conclusions

When the 11 local authorities were contacted in 1995 only a few could supply figures for pregnant young women or young parents who were currently being looked after. Others admitted that no systematic recording took place although the numbers were thought to be high. In some ways this lack of data is not surprising as young people can move in and out of the care system quickly. However, the lack of data is of concern as it reflected the lack of a planning base.

We have explored the issues around preparation and support for parenthood predominantly from the viewpoint of young people, the majority of whom were living in residential care. It was not our intention to exclude foster care and we have tried to draw on the previous experiences of foster care that many young people had. Nevertheless our conclusions must be seen to relate primarily to the views and experiences of young people looked after by local authorities in a residential setting.

Drawing together the available evidence we should not wish to conclude that being looked after automatically equates with or leads to an increased likelihood of becoming pregnant. Some young people enter public care because they are pregnant (though others leave for the same reason); there is evidence that family conflict is linked with teenage pregnancies and our two samples in component 2 were not matched for levels of conflict within the family. Efforts were made to match by sex, gender and age, and, to a lesser extent, social class. Social class in itself, however, is not an indicator of conflict and therefore the looked after young people may be no different from those in wider community who have also experienced family disruption. We can infer from some responses that the looked after young people's perspective of family life incorporated both arguments and violence and that this perspective was not shared by the non-looked after young people.

However, there are ways in which the care system seems to compound some problems and fails to alleviate others.

Living in residential care would appear to place extra pressure on young women *and* young men to embark on sexual relationships at a relatively early age and provide them with an enhanced opportunity to do so.

Looked after young people do not seem to benefit from positive relationships with adults from which they might learn. Parents and social workers were seen as being prone to ignore them, disregard their feelings and opinions, and make decisions on their behalf without consulting them. Young people are not afforded the opportunity to learn about trust and respect and, feeling unloved and uncared for, might be more likely to enter into a relationship without consideration of either the suitability of the partner or the implications of their actions than would those who possess more confidence in themselves. Unless they receive affection and learn to understand the nature of that which is not contingent upon sex they are likely to continue in their search for love through sexual relationships and parenthood.

Young people in public care aspire to have access to education, training and employment in the future in the same way that those not in public care do, but they look just as much to early marriage and parenting, to a far greater extent than their peers. We do not know whether this is hedging their bets, wanting everything, or being unrealistic about what can be achieved in the late teens but it suggests a need for help with planning the future.

Because young people in public care do not usually participate in decisions made about them and because such decisions are often made on a temporary basis at short notice they have developed a fore-shortened view of the future and a fatalistic acceptance of life. It is, therefore, difficult for them to see the implications of embarking on sexual relationships and even more difficult for them to see the long-term consequences of pregnancy. They do not make decisions when unintended conceptions occur for a variety of reasons, but one of them is because no one helps them to. The appropriate intervention may be counselling, advice, therapy or simply being given information and support. Currently there appears to be nothing.

It would appear from our study that teenagers in general might benefit from a further reinforcement of the need not only to obtain but also to use contraception if they do not wish to be pregnant. But for looked after young people such messages go only part way to changing their patterns of behaviour. Equally, if not more, important for them are understanding relationships, resisting unwelcome pressure and, crucially, having their emotional needs addressed. These require a coordinated approach and the long-term investment of resources.

Boys and young men who are looked after appear to receive more pressure from girls to have sex than do their counterparts who are not looked after. At the same time, because of their lack of concern for the consequences of their actions and their discomfort in discussing contraception, they are unlikely to see prevention of pregnancy as a priority. They are even more likely than looked after girls to aspire to be married and have children at an early age. Yet little attention is paid to the sex education of young men looked after, and even less to their emotional needs. It might prove profitable to amend the common perception that preventing teenage pregnancy implies a focus on girls and young women.

Local authorities must accept that the young people whom they look after will have sexual relationships and should equip those who work with them with policies, guidelines and training that will allow them to work confidently with these young people to ensure that they are appropriately protected from undesired relationships and unwanted pregnancies.

When young women do become pregnant and choose to have the baby there should be procedures and services in place to ensure the best possible outcome for the mother and her baby. These should include continuing support, the provision for her education and a variety of accommodation to suit her age and needs and which takes into account the nature of her relationship with the baby's father.

References

Acheson, D (chair) (1998) *Independent Inquiry into Health Inequalities*. The Stationery Office

Action on Aftercare Consortium (1996) *Too Much Too Young: The failure of social policy in meeting the needs of care leavers*. Barnardo's

Alderson, P (1995) *Listening to Children: Children, ethics and social research*. Barnardo's

Allen, I (1987) *Education in Sex and Personal Relationships*. Policy Studies Institute

Allen, I (1991) *Family Planning and Pregnancy Counselling Projects for Young People*. Policy Studies Institute

Audit Commission (1994) *Seen But Not Heard*. HMSO

Babb, P (1994) 'Teenage conceptions and fertility in England and Wales, 1971–1991', *Population Trends*, 74, 12–17

Balding, J (1994) *Young People in 1993*. Exeter University, Schools Health Education Unit

Balding, J (1995) *Young People in 1994*. Exeter University, Schools Health Education Unit

Baldo, M, Aggleton, P and Slutkin, E (1993) *Does Sex Education Lead to Earlier or Increased Sexual Activity in Youth?* Report PO-D02-3444, World Health Organisation

Bartley, M and others (1994) 'Birth weight and later socioeconomic disadvantage: evidence from the 1958 British cohort study', *British Medical Journal*, 309, 1475–8

Bebbington, J and Miles, A (1989) 'Children who enter local authority care', *British Journal of Social Work,* 19, 5, 349–68

Berridge, D and Brodie, I (1997) *Children's Homes Revisited*. Jessica Kingsley

Biehal, N and others (1992) *Prepared for Living? A survey of young people leaving the care of the local authorities*. National Children's Bureau

Biehal, N and others (1994) 'Leaving care in England: a research perspective', *Children and Youth Services Review,* 16, 3/4, 231–54

Biehal, N and others (1995) *Moving On: Young people and leaving care schemes*. HMSO

Bonnerjea, L (1990) *Leaving Care in London*. London Boroughs Children's Regional Planning Committee

Botting, B, Rosato, M and Wood, R (1998) 'Teenage mothers and the health of their children', *Population Trends*, 93, 19–28

Boyer, D and Fine, M (1992) 'Sexual abuse as a factor in adolescent pregnancy and child maltreatment', *Family Planning Perspectives*, 24, 1, 4–11

Bradburn, NM 'Response effects' *in* Rossi, P, Wright, J and Anderson, A *eds* (1983) *Handbook of Survey Research*. New York: Academic Press

Brannen J and others (1994) *Young People, Health and Family Life*. Open University Press

Bremner, J and Hillin, J (1993) *Sexuality, Young People and Care*. Central Council for Education and Training in Social Work

Broad, B (1994) *Leaving Care in the 1990s: The results of a national survey*. Royal Philanthropic Society

Bromham, DR and Cartmill, RSV (1993) 'Are current sources of contraceptive advice adequate to meet changes in contraceptive practice? A study of patients requesting termination of pregnancy', *British Journal of Family Planning*, 19, 2, 179–83

Brook Advisory Centres (1995) *Annual Report*. Brook Advisory Centres

Brook, SJ and Smith, C (1991) 'Do combined oral contraceptive users know how to take the pill correctly?', *British Journal of Family Planning*, 17, 1, 18–20

Buchanan, A and others (1993) *Answering Back: Report by young people being looked after on The Children Act 1989*. Southampton University, Department of Social Work

Bullock, R, Little, M and Millham, S (1993) *Going Home*. Dartmouth

Burghes, B, Clarke, L and Cronin, N (1997) *Fathers and Fatherhood in Britain*. Occasional paper 23, Family Policy Studies Centre

Burghes, L and Brown, M (1995) *Single Lone Mothers: Problems, Prospects and Policies*. Family Policy Studies Centre

Cartwright, A (1988) 'Unintended pregnancy that leads to babies', *Social Science and Medicine*, 27, 249–54

Cleaver, H (1996) *Focus on Teenagers: Research into practice*. HMSO

Coleman, J and Dennison, C (1998) 'Teenage parenthood', *Children and Society*, 12, 4, 306–14

Combes, G and Schonveld, A (1992) *Life Will Never Be The Same Again*. Health Education Authority

Corlyon, J and McGuire, C (1997) *Young Parents in Public Care: Pregnancy and parenthood among young people looked after by local authorities*. National Children's Bureau

Coyne, AM (no date) *School-girl Mothers*. Health Education Authority

Dawson, N (1996) 'Report on the 1994 survey of educational provision for pregnant school-girl and school-girl mothers', *Journal of Adolescent Health and Welfare*, 9, 1, 12–24

Dawson, N (1997) 'The provision of education and opportunities for future employment for pregnant schoolgirls and schoolgirl mothers in the UK', *Children and Society*, 11, 252–63

Department for Education and Employment (1997) *Excellence in Schools*. Stationery Office

Department of Health (1991a) *Children in the Public Care*. HMSO

Department of Health (1991b) *The Children Act 1989: Guidance and Regulations. Volume 4 Residential Care*. HMSO

Department of Health (1991c) *The Children Act 1989: Guidance and Regulations. Volume 3 Family Placements*. HMSO

Department of Health (1991d) *Looking After Children: A guide to the action and assessment schedules*. HMSO

Department of Health (1992) *The Health of the Nation: A strategy for health in England*. HMSO

Department of Health (1995a) *The Education of Children Who Are Looked After by Local Authorities*. Department of Health Social Services Inspectorate

Department of Health (1995b) *Looking After Children: Action and Assessment Schedules*. HMSO

Department of Health and Department for Education and Employment (1996) *Children's Services Planning: Guidance*, LAC(96)10. Department of Health and Department for Education and Employment

Department of Health (1997a) *"...When Leaving Home is Leaving Care..." An Inspection of Services for Young People Leaving Care*. Department of Health Social Services Inspectorate

Department of Health (1997b) *Children Looked After by Local Authorities. Year Ending 31 March 1996*. HMSO

Department of Health (1998a) *Quality Protects: Framework for action*. The Stationery Office

Department of Health (1998b) *Our Healthier Nation: A contract for health*. The Stationery Office

Department of Social Security (1998) *New Ambitions for Our Country: A New Contract for Welfare*, Cm3805. The Stationery Office

Dryfoos, J (1990) *Adolescents at Risk: Prevalence and prevention*. Oxford University Press

Duncan, G and others (1990) 'Termination of pregnancy: lessons for prevention', *British Journal of Family Planning*, 15, 112–17

Education Act 1993. HMSO

Fleissig, A (1991) 'Unintended pregnancies and the use of contraception: changes from 1984 to 1989', *British Medical Journal,* 302, 6769, 147

Ford, N (1991) *The Socio-sexual Lifestyles of Young People in South West England*. University of Exeter

Furstenburg, F, Brooks-Gunn, J and Morgan, SP (1987) *Adolescent Mothers in Later Life*. Cambridge University Press

Garcia J, France-Dawson M and Macfarlane, A (1994) *Improving Infant Health*. Health Education Authority

Garnett, L (1992) *Leaving Care and After.* National Children's Bureau

Gough, D (1964) Paper presented at International Congress of Psychotherapy

Grunseit, A and Kippax, S (1994) *Effects of Sex Education on Young People's Sexual Behaviour.* Geneva: World Health Organisation

Hazel, N (1996) 'Elicitation techniques with young people', *Social Research Update*, 12, University of Surrey

Health Education Authority (1996) *Health in England 1995*. Office of Population Censuses and Surveys

Health Education Authority (1998) *Reducing the Rate of Teenage Conceptions. Towards a national programme*. Draft document for consultation. Health Education Authority

Hirst, J (1994) *Not in Front of the Grown Ups: a study of the social and sexual lives of 15 and 16 year-olds*. Publications

Hoinville, G and Jowell, R (1980) *Survey Research Practice*. Heinemann

Holland, J, Mauthner, M and Sharpe, S (1996) *Family Matters: Communicating health messages in the family*. Health Education Authority

Home Office Ministerial Group on the Family (1998) *Supporting Families*. The Stationery Office

Hope, P and Sharland, P (1997) *Tomorrow's Parents. Developing parenthood education in schools*. Calouste Gulbenkian Foundation

Houghton, A (1994) 'Knowledge of contraception among abortion seekers and non-pregnant women', *British Journal of Family Planning*, 20, 69–72

House of Commons (1998) *Children Looked After by Local Authorities,* Health Committee Second Report. The Stationery Office

Hudson, F and Ineichen, B (1991) *Taking It Lying Down: Sexuality and teenage motherhood*. Macmillan

Institute of Housing (1993) *One Parent Families – Are They Jumping the Housing Queue?* Institute of Housing

Johnson, A and others (1994) *Sexual Attitudes and Lifestyles.* Blackwell Scientific Publications

Jones, EF and others (1985) 'Teenage pregnancy in developed countries: determinants and policy implications', *Family Planning Perspectives,* 17, 2, 53–63

Jones, G (1987) 'Leaving the parental home: an analysis of early housing careers', *Journal of Social Policy,* 16, 1, 49–74

Kiernan, K (1995) *Transition to Parenthood: Young mothers, young fathers – associated factors and later life experiences.* Joseph Rowntree Foundation

Krueger, RA (1994) *Focus Groups: A practical guide for applied research.* Sage

Lalond, S (1995) 'Teenage dads', *New Generation,* June, 9

Lee, R (1993) *Doing Research on Sensitive Topics.* Sage

Leigh, B (1990) 'The relationship between substance use during sex to high-risk sex behaviour', *Journal of Sex Research,* 27, 199–213

McGuire, C and Corlyon, J (1997) *Health Promotion and Looked After Children in Brent and Harrow.* National Children's Bureau

McRae, S (1993) *Cohabiting Mothers.* Policy Studies Institute

Makinson, C (1985) 'The health consequences of teenage fertility', *Family Planning Perspectives,* 17, 3, 132–9

Marsh, P (1996) 'Child care', *Research Matters,* 2, 60–2

Marsh, P and Crow, G (1998) *Family Group Conferences in Child Welfare.* Blackwell Science

Mason, J and Lewis, H (1999) *Time to Decide: A guide to support young people in public care who need to make decisions about pregnancy.* National Children's Bureau

Mellanby, A, Phelps, F and Tripp, JH (1993) 'Teenagers, sex and risk taking', *British Medical Journal,* 307, 6895, 25

Meyrick, J and Harris, R (1995) 'Adolescent sexual behaviour, contraceptive use and pregnancy: a review', *Association for Child Psychology and Psychiatry Review and Newsletter,* 16, 5, 245–51

Moore, S and Rosenthal, D (1993) *Sexuality in Adolescence.* Routledge

Mori (1991) *Young Adults: health lifestyles.* Health Education Authority

Musick, J (1993) *Young, Poor and Pregnant: The psychology of teenage motherhood.* US, New Haven: Yale University Press

National Foster Care Association (1994) *Choosing to Foster: The challenge to care.* National Foster Care Association

National Health Service Centre for Reviews and Dissemination (1997) 'Preventing and reducing the adverse effects of unintended teenage pregnancies', *Effective Health Care,* 3, 1

NFER/HEA (1993) *A Survey of Health Education Policies in Schools.* Health Education Authority

Office for National Statistics (1998a) *Birth Statistics,* Series FMI, 26. The Stationery Office

Office for National Statistics (1998b) *Conceptions in England and Wales 1996,* Monitor FM1/98/1. The Stationery Office

Office for Population Censuses Surveys (1992) *Birth Statistics,* Series FMI, 19. HMSO

Office for Population Censuses Surveys (1995) *General Household Survey 1993.* HMSO

Office for Population Censuses Surveys (1997) *Mortality Statistics. Childhood, infant and perinatal. England and Wales.* Stationery Office

Osofsky, J, Hann, D and Peebles, C 'Adolescent parenthood: risks and opportunities for parents and infants' *in* Zeannah, C ed. (1993) *Handbook of Infant Mental Health.* New York: Guilford Press

Parker, R and others (1991) *Assessing Outcomes in Child Care*. The Report of an Independent Working Party established by the Department of Health. HMSO

Patel-Kanwal, H and Frances Lenderyou, G (1998) *Let's Talk About Sex and Relationships. A policy framework for working with looked after children and young people*. National Children's Bureau

Pawlby, SJ, Mills, A and Quinton, D (1997) 'Vulnerable adolescent girls: opposite-sex relationships', *Journal of Psychology and Psychiatry*, 38, 8, 909–20

Phoenix, A (1991) *Young Mothers?* Polity Press

Polnay, L (1994) *Children in Community Homes. Health, mental health and health promotion needs*. Unpublished paper

Pugh, G, De'Ath, E and Smith, C (1994) *Confident Parents, Confident Children*. National Children's Bureau

Quinton, D, and others (1993) 'Partners, peers and pathways: assortative pairing and continuities in conduct disorder', *Development and Psychopathology*, 5, 763–83

Roberts, H and Sachdev, D (1996) *Young People's Social Attitudes: Having their say – the views of 12–19 year-olds*. Barnardo's

Rudat, K, Speed, M and Ryan, H (1992) *Tomorrow's Young Adults: 9–15-year-olds look at drugs, exercise and smoking*. Health Education Authority

Rutter, M (1974) 'Dimensions of parenthood: some myths and some suggestions', *The Family in Society, Dimensions of Parenthood*. HMSO

Selman, P (1998) 'Teenage fertility, poverty and the welfare debate in the United States and Europe', paper presented at Committee for International Cooperation in National Research in Demography seminar, *Poverty, Fertility and Family Planning*, Mexico City, 2–4 June 1998

Sex Education Forum (1992a) *A Framework for School Sex Education*. National Children's Bureau

Shaw, C and The Who Cares? Trust (1998) *Remember My Messages*. The Who Cares? Trust

Simpson, B, McCarthy, P and Walker, J (1995) Being There: Fathers after divorce. Relate Centre for Family Studies

Simms, M and Smith, C (1986) *Teenage Mothers and their Partners*. HMSO

Sinclair, R, Garnett, L and Berridge, D (1995) *Social Work and Assessment with Adolescents*. National Children's Bureau

Skuse, T (1995) *Residential Care for Young Mothers: A guide for staff training*. Trust for the Study of Adolescence, Brighton

Speak, S, Cameron, S and Gilroy, R (1997) *Young Single Fathers: Participation in fatherhood – barriers and bridges*. Family Policy Studies Centre and Joseph Rowntree Foundation

Speak, S and others (1995) *Young Single Mothers: Barriers to independent living*. Family Policies Study Centre

Stacey, M (1990) *The Sociology of Health and Healing*. Routledge

Sweeting, H and West, P (1995) 'Family life and health in adolescence: a role for culture in the health inequalities debate?', *Social Science and Medicine,* 40, 2, 163–75

Tabberer, S and others (1998) *Teenage Pregnancy and Choice: A summary of interim findings* Studies Unit, Anglia Polytechnic University

Thomson, R and Scott, L (1991) *Learning About Sex: Young women and the social construction of sexual identity*. Tufnell Press

Thomson, R and Scott, L (1992) An Enquiry into Sex Education: Report of a survey into local education authority support and monitoring of school sex education. National Children's Bureau

Triseliotis, J and others (1995) *Teenagers and Social Work Services*. HMSO

Utting, W (1997) *People Like Us*. The Stationery Office

Ward, H ed. (1995) *Looking After Children: Research into practice*. HMSO

Wellings, K and others (1994) *Social Behaviour in Britain. The national survey of sexual attitudes and lifestyles.* Penguin

Wilson, W (1994) *Lone Parents and Housing*, Research Paper 94/11 House of Commons Library

Appendix A: Research design, methods and sampling

This appendix offers further information on sampling and methods employed in the project and additional details on the samples in the two components.

Sampling considerations

Component 1

Component 1 of the project aimed to look at the support offered to pregnant young women and young parents in the care of local authorities. In 1996 there were just over 14,000 girls aged ten years of age and over in the care of local authorities (Department of Health, 1997b). It was assumed that in any one local authority the number of young pregnant women or young mothers was likely to be low and consequently young women who had or were expecting babies *either* while they were being *or* shortly after they ceased to be looked after were included in the sample.

In the selection of young parents or mothers-to-be it was hoped that their age, gender, parental status (parents or mother-to-be), type of placement, and length of time looked after could be considered. However, it was by no means certain that any selection would be possible, partly because local authorities themselves might be unsure of how many pregnant young women or young parents they were looking after, and partly because of young people's movement in and out of the care system. In the event no selection was possible.

Component 2

In conducting the quantitative research with the looked after young people and their peers in component 2, it was considered that the age band interviewed should be relatively narrow so that in theory all young people included should have reached a similar stage in the National Curriculum.

A major aspect of the study was young people's expectations of the future and it was considered advantageous to assess these at a time when the young people were not focused on public examinations and the manner in which success or failure in these might influence their decisions and expectations. In the comparator sample to be drawn from schools it was also circumspect to avoid seeking access to year 11 classes which would be heavily focused on preparation for public examinations.

Consequently it was decided to focus on 14–15-year-olds since this age group would have sufficient knowledge of the issues involved (such as pregnancy and contraception), be starting to form views independently of adults and be considering their future, yet not too preoccupied with the external examination system. They would also be on the brink of making decisions about service usage independently: a study by Brannen and others (1994) suggested that young people are most likely to make unaccompanied visits to their general practitioner around the age of 15–16 years.

Description of methods

Component 1

Sampling procedures

In deciding in which local authorities to base the study several factors were taken into account:

- Locality. The aim was to obtain a geographical spread while minimising travel between authorities.
- The size and type of local authorities. A mix of metropolitan, city and county councils, if possible avoiding those scheduled for re-organisation during the study period, was seen as ideal.
- Ethnic composition. Some authorities with a high proportion of minority ethnic groups, especially Black African and Black Caribbean people whose children show an over-representation in care statistics, were to be included.
- The rates of children being looked after by local authorities (rate per 1000 under 18-year-olds) and percentages in residential care. Authorities with higher rates of looked after children were to be chosen if possible, in order to maximise the population size.

Additional criteria used to guide the initial selection of the areas included the stipulation that the local authorities in question should have shown an initial interest in the research by proactively contacting the research team or by simply being members of NCB. Given the way in which young people were to be contacted, cooperation from each social services department was key. Approaching members of NCB – and nearly all local authorities are members – was seen as a way of ensuring more collaborative working arrangements from the start. This may, however, have excluded local authorities with different practices regarding looked after young people.

On this basis four broad areas of the country, north-east, north-west, central and south, each containing several local authorities, were chosen. Estimating how many local authorities to approach was problematical not only in terms of their response but also because of the difficulty in establishing how many young people in any authority would be relevant to this piece of research. Once the approval of the Association of Directors of Social Services had been given, a letter was sent to the director of social services in each authority outlining the research and inviting participation. Agreement was obtained from, and it was decided to proceed with the research in, 11 authorities: two in the north-east, four in the north-west, two in the central area and three in the south. The characteristics and statistics relating to each of these authorities appear in a previous publication (Corlyon and McGuire, 1997). Although the original intention was to base the study in four or five authorities it was considered appropriate at this stage to include more than that number in view of the uncertainty about numbers of looked after young women who were pregnant or parents within the authorities.

The findings concerning local authority policy and practice cannot be taken as representative. In addition, at the time of interview many local authorities were already considering changing their approach to issues of sexual health and looked after children; thus the findings cannot be taken as indicative of the current situation, rather as illustrative of why change is necessary.

Methods and data collection

Contact with the relevant young people was made by social workers or carers who forwarded a letter from us explaining the research to young people who met the criteria for selection. It was agreed that young people would be invited to participate but that no pressure would be put on them to do so. After the initial contact, no reminder letters would be sent. The young people who were agreeable to interview chose either to return the form that had been enclosed with the letter directly to the researcher (as the majority did) or to ask the social worker to establish contact on their behalf.

The fact that we were dependent on 'gatekeepers' (social workers and carers) for access to respondents had advantages and disadvantages. Some social workers not only forwarded the letter but also discussed the research with potential respondents which greatly facilitated our task. Conversely others were often selective in forwarding letters and used their judgement and knowledge of the young people concerned in deciding whom to approach on our behalf. Further, in view of their heavy workload and more pressing concerns, the research may have been given a low priority by some of our link people. Young people came forward for interview in areas where gatekeepers showed most interest in the research.

Once an agreement for interview had been received, contact was immediately made with the young person and a meeting arranged. A reminder letter was sent to arrive the day before the scheduled meeting. Arranged meetings were frequently forgotten by young people and, though always successfully re-arranged, presented resource implications.

Interviews lasted for amounts of time varying between one and three hours depending on factors such as the loquaciousness of the young person and the extent of interruptions: since most of the interviews were conducted with babies or young children present they were inevitably stopped and started several times. Respondents generally appeared to welcome the opportunity to talk about their experiences.

The interview schedule for young people covered six topics: background, education, sexual relations, pregnancy and parenthood, transition out of care and a final general section covering attitudes and aspirations.

Corresponding schedules for carers and social workers covered background information on the young person, their education, transition out of care and a general section on her support and future needs. These interviews always took place after those with the young person. They typically lasted between half an hour and an hour; their duration was often dictated by the amount of time a worker could make available.

After extending the data collection period for as long as possible without delaying the agreed timescale of the research, 30 interviews with young people and 20 with their social workers or carers were completed. This was lower than the target number. In addition to reasons connected to gatekeepers and re-arranged visits set out above, other factors that influenced the number were that young fathers were particularly difficult to identify and, once identified, apparently extremely reluctant to agree to an interview; and many young women, in particular those who are very young, who become pregnant while being accommodated return to live with their family or friends and their involvement with the social services department ends.

Component 2

Sampling procedures

The population of interest for this quantitative stage of the project was young people aged 14–15 years, with samples drawn from the looked after population and from their peers in the wider community. The intention was to achieve a sample of 200 for each group with approximately 50 per cent males and 50 per cent females.

Looked after sample

A sampling frame of looked after children does not exist nationally and, were it to be available, the logistics of completing a survey across a number of areas would have had resource implications beyond this study. Having successfully worked with a number of local authorities in the first part of the study, it was decided to conduct this second part in a small number of these. It was estimated that three to four areas might generate a sufficient sample.

The research team already had some knowledge about which local authorities had accessible and comprehensive lists of looked after young people and the intention was to approach each of these areas in turn to ask for additional help. However, two factors affected the decision on how many areas were approached. Firstly, as we describe later, the fieldwork took much longer than expected with the result that the target sample size was reduced to 100. Secondly, the first area approached generated almost all of the respondents on which the analysis is based, and only one additional area was approached. The quality of the list provided was such that young people of the correct age could be identified, as could the placement type (foster or residential care).

In effect there was no need for a sampling strategy since it was theoretically possible to contact all young people (165) on the list provided. However, because of the speed at which some placements change and some young people move into and out of the public care system, lists soon date, and from this first list 82 young people could not be traced. A further 11 were located in residential schools or secure units outside the area and there were four refusals from either a parent or a social worker. The potential sample was, therefore, 68 young people who were invited to attend one of five meetings organised for completing the questionnaire. Of these, 21 attended and filled in the questionnaire and a further 18 who had been unable to attend one of the meetings but who had shown an interest in the research subsequently completed a questionnaire. A second list was drawn seven months later which contained 102 names, 27 of which had been on the previous list. There were three refusals by social workers and a further ten young people had moved placement or returned home, leaving a potential sample size of 62. On this occasion individual visits were made to residential and foster homes which resulted in a further 51 questionnaires being completed, some by young people from the first list who had not attended the meetings.

In the second area sampling was more problematic. The list contained 42 names: four were in placements outside the area, seven had moved or returned home, there were six refusals from parents, social workers or carers. This left a potential sample size of 25 of whom 16 completed questionnaires.

In total 106 young people completed questionnaires. From a potential sample size of 155 this represented a response rate of 68 per cent which was highly satisfactory given the nature of the sample and justified the extra resources that had been invested in collecting the quantitative data. Had we been dependent on a postal questionnaire, the outcome would not have been so good. A recent postal survey of young people aged eight to 20 who are looked after resulted in 2073 usable questionnaires being returned from the 45,000 that were distributed (Shaw and The Who Cares? Trust, 1998). Moreover, because our method involved a researcher always being on hand to help or to answer queries, the quality of the data was very good.

Response rate

Total names supplied	282
Unable to contact (discharged from care, moved placement, no address outside placement)	114
Parent refused or social worker considered unsuitable	13
Potential sample	**155**
Written refusals from young people	14
Unable to arrange visit or appointment not kept	35
Questionnaires completed	106
Rate	**68%**

The original intention was to complete the collection of quantitative data and then select, from those who had completed a questionnaire, a sample for the qualitative interview. However, given that young people frequently change placement, decisions on sampling became problematic and a decision was taken to interview those who had given their agreement as soon as possible after the questionnaire was filled in (typically one or two weeks later). Personal or group interviews took place with 38 of these young people.

A major drawback of the looked after sample was that, despite consistent efforts to make it otherwise, the sample mainly comprised young people in residential care.

School sample

The original intention had been to collect data from young people aged 14–15 years who were not looked after to match data collected from those who were in public care.

A decision was taken to contact this sample in schools. The disadvantage of this approach is that the sample excludes pupils not in school, for example those excluded, truanting or ill. This was addressed in part by including a small sample drawn from a local youth club.

Given that the aim was to compare the two groups in terms of attitudes to the future and to parenthood, it was decided that the school sample should be selected to match the looked after sample as far as possible so that the findings would not be confounded by issues associated with class or better levels of education.

Two issues central to the decision making about the school sample were which variables should be matched and the resources to locate suitable cases.

Taking the latter point first, a decision was made not to match by individual cases. It was considered that resources did not permit such an exercise. The groups would be matched by general socio-demographic variables. It was believed that religion might also be important given the subject of the survey. The selection of variables was problematic. Age and gender were obvious choices, followed by social class. However, establishing the latter was likely to be difficult since:

- In their analysis of birth weight and socioeconomic disadvantage, Bartley and others (1994) argued that social class alone is unsatisfactory as an indicator of disadvantage in childhood. As a larger number of people spend time out of the labour force, usual occupation is less reliable as an indicator of living standards.
- Individuals in the looked after sample might have little contact with their parents and judging occupation may be difficult. As it transpired, a large number of them claimed to have little contact with their father if not both parents, and in the pilot stage of the questionnaire the majority of young people objected to the inclusion of questions about their parents.

A decision was taken to match by general **area profile.** Other attempts at comparing community groups of children with those in contact with social services departments have also adopted a broad approach to matching. For example, Pawlby, Mills and Quinton (1997) matched by areas comparable in socioeconomic level to the borough from which the 'high-risk' group was drawn; in evaluating the *Looking After Children* materials random samples were taken from selected schools and supplemented with snowballing techniques (Ward, 1995).

However, matching by area presented difficulties, too. Firstly, looked after children interviewed in residential care homes were often drawn from across a wide area of the city. Secondly, the schools selected also drew their school population from outside the wards in which they were located. Thirdly, the researcher was to a great extent dependent on local knowledge of areas, schools and willingness of school staff to engage in survey work.

The directors of education were contacted in each of the two areas where interviewing of the looked after population took place. Sampling proceeded in the one area from which a reply was obtained. Using local professional knowledge of schools, three were selected as possible matches; it was anticipated that these would be sufficient to generate the reduced target of

106 interviews. Additionally, again using local knowledge and contacts, a small sample was drawn for a youth club.

The sample for the qualitative interviews was not matched with that for the looked after sample, but rather included all those young people who were willing to participate, who numbered 29 in total.

Methods and data collection

When the fieldwork was initiated there were few available surveys of the looked after population from which lessons could be learnt regarding sampling and methods. Marsh (1996), in his study of young people leaving the care system, had obtained a high response rate but neither the method nor the target sample was comparable to our own. Problems of contacting young people for interview had been experienced in a study evaluating social work services for teenagers (Triseliotis and others, 1995). Towards the end of this project, a study comparing young women known to social services with a matched sample from the wider community was published (Pawlby, Mills and Quinton, 1997).

However, the research team did benefit from the body of research that has been undertaken among young people in general in recent years. A number of questionnaires were collected and examined in terms of construction and content; for example, those used in *Tomorrow's Young Adults* (Rudat, Speed and Ryan, 1992); *Young People in 1994* (Balding, 1995); the *Trent Health Lifestyle Young People's Survey*; *Young People's Attitudes* (Roberts and Sachdev, 1996); *European Network for Health Promoting Schools* (NFER); and the *Sex and Lifestyle Questionnaire* (Medical Research Council Medical Sociology Unit). With permission of the relevant researchers, original questions were used or adapted for use here. Questions considered to be particularly sensitive, for example those on abortion, were addressed by introducing vignettes (Hazel, 1996) or by phrasing questions on the topics of sex and early parenthood in general rather than in a personal terms, for example 'Do young people feel ... ?' This is considered to be a helpful method in aiding responses (Hoinville and Jowell, 1980; Bradburn, 1983).

Given the resources available for the survey a self-completion questionnaire was decided upon. Initially there were concerns about literacy among the intended sample. For this reason the number of open-ended questions was kept to a minimum, as it was thought that writing might be more problematical than reading. Most young people successfully completed the questionnaire in about 40 minutes. Help was available when they experienced difficulties.

The questionnaire was filled in during a PSE lesson or form period in the three schools visited and during an early evening session at the youth club. As described above and in Chapter 1, collecting the information from looked after young people was more problematic, although ultimately successful.

The outcropping approach to sampling that was adopted in area two and in the second wave of data collection in area one is a cost-effective approach to sampling, but its disadvantage lies in ignoring isolated cases (Lee, 1993), which in this case included young people in foster care who were contacted on a one to one basis, although far from successfully. Attempts to meet individually with those in foster care resulted in five questionnaires being completed. The usual scenario was that telephone numbers were not available and no written response was received from either young people or their carers.

Because of the complexities of collecting the data a smaller than anticipated sample size was achieved. In total 265 questionnaires were completed: 106 among looked after young people and 159 among the school sample. Male respondents were over-represented in the latter sample which was, therefore, reduced to match the looked after sample by discarding a proportion of responses from males along with a small number of spoiled or substantially incomplete questionnaires.

Consent

Once the list of the looked after young people had been received, a letter was sent to the social workers identified on the list asking whether they were agreeable to the named persons participating in the research if they wished to do so. If there were no objections a letter was sent to the young people giving a brief outline of the research and the nature of their involvement should they choose to participate. They were asked to send back a form (a stamped addressed envelope was included) if they did not wish to be involved further. Social workers were asked to forward a letter to parents explaining the nature of the research, seeking parental approval and inviting them to contact the researcher if they wanted more information. Letters were sent to foster carers and managers of residential units with information about the research and the potential involvement of the young people and an undertaking to keep them informed of all contacts with the young people.

Those young people who had not declined further involvement and whose parents or social workers had not refused on their behalf were contacted again to arrange to meet. In the first wave in area one this was to invite them to one of the organised meetings in the area where they lived. Subsequently this contact was to arrange a visit to the residential home or to the foster home. Where possible this was done first by telephone and then followed up by a letter of confirmation designed to arrive the day before the proposed visit.

In the school sample the name of a contact teacher in each school was supplied. He or she sought the permission and cooperation of other staff where appropriate. Letters were sent to the contact teacher for distribution to pupils and their parents. The teacher arranged the times for visits to the school to complete the questionnaires and subsequent visits for interviews and group discussions with those pupils who had indicated their willingness to take part in the qualitative study.

Sample details

Component I

In terms of their care history, the young women fell into two distinct groups: those who had first been looked after in childhood and had not returned to their families of origin (just over one third of the sample) and those who had first been looked after in adolescence. Other research has pointed to the relatively high numbers of young people who begin to be looked after in their teenage years, especially in the age range of 14–17 (Garnett, 1992; Biehal and others, 1994).

Looked after in adolescence

Those in the larger group who had begun to be looked after as adolescents typically did so at the age of 14 and the vast majority were being accommodated under Section 20 of the Children Act 1989. Only two young women stated that there was, or had been, a care order in effect and in both cases they had begun to be looked after at the age of 13 because of sexual abuse by one of their family.

Only two had had a previous episode of being accommodated and in both cases this was at the age of 12; they had then returned home for a period of time before being looked after again at the age of 14 when both were pregnant. The pregnancy was given as a contributing factor for their re-entry into the care system. In only one case, a 15-year-old, was the pregnancy stated to be the sole reason for the young woman no longer being able to live with her family.

The most common reason given for becoming accommodated at this age was family breakdown, in most cases the young woman failing to get on with parents; this was usually with the mother and, very often, the mother's new partner. The presence of the new partner was doubly disadvantageous since it not only led to the young woman being looked after in the first place but also jeopardized her chances of subsequently resuming a good relationship with her mother.

In two cases, where the young woman had been living with both parents, her relationship with a boyfriend was a pressing reason for her being looked after. In one of these cases the young woman considered it was because her boyfriend was not white and her parents were racist.

In more than half the cases the decision to become looked after was stated to be either solely at the young woman's request or a joint decision with her parent or parents. The exceptions were the two who had a care order, the three who were already pregnant and one other whose mother asked for her daughter to be looked after overnight as a punishment because she was unable to control her behaviour. The result in this case was a rapid deterioration in behaviour, pregnancy and an extended period of being looked after.

Five young women came from families where the parents had been living together at the time when they became looked after. With one exception the other young women from these families had, at the time of interview, good relationships with their parents who were helpful and supportive in many respects. In the remaining case, in which religion was a major factor, the young woman continued to have no contact with either parent.

Only one young woman had no siblings: the remainder came from families of varying size and composition, several of which included step-siblings and/or half-siblings. Their own position in the family appeared to have little bearing on whether or not the young woman became looked after. Only two had siblings who were also looked after and one had an older brother who had left home at an early age and who, at the time of the interview, was thought to be in prison.

A characteristic of this group of young women was a reported high level of unhappiness. In some cases, especially amongst those in their later teens, this manifested itself as a current dissatisfaction with certain aspects of their life. However, other young women referred to previous bouts of depression, self-harm and attempted suicide. Since questions on mental health were not asked and this information was volunteered, it is possible that many others in the sample were likewise troubled. Similarly, and possibly connected, was the voluntary disclosure of domestic abuse against them. More than half of the respondents in this group mentioned that some kind of ill treatment had featured in their lives. In addition to the two young women who had been sexually abused at home, others mentioned mental abuse from parents and violence from mothers' new partners and from their own partners. None referred to abuse from carers.

This group did not, overall, appear to have suffered excessively frequent changes of placement. Several had progressed smoothly from residential care in a children's home to an independent living unit. Those who had been placed in foster care appeared to have experienced a larger number of placement moves.

Looked after since childhood

The smaller group of young women who had first been looked after in childhood were different from the group described above in several respects. The majority of them were being looked after due to their mother's inability or unwillingness to care for them. None came from two-parent families: either one parent had died or the parents had separated, and usually a new partner was involved. In some cases the arrival of a new partner had meant that the parent had had to make a choice and the children had been the losers. One young woman related that her mother had left home to live with a new partner leaving her and her two siblings with their father. When he, too, found a new partner he asked for the children to be looked after by social services and had had very little contact with them since. In another case the young woman's mother went to live abroad with her new partner and the children were dispersed to various schools and foster carers.

Apart from the very small number of cases where a parent had requested social services' involvement, the majority of young women were looked after under the terms of a care order. Moreover, most of them came from families in which at least one other sibling was also being looked after: often the children from one relationship were looked after while those from a parent's subsequent relationship were not.

Because they had spent much longer in the care system than the group above, they were much more likely to have experienced changes of placement. They were also more likely to have had a placement with foster carers. In our sample the highest number of foster placements reported by any one person was 25 along with 'a few' residential placements in a 16-year care career. Other young women had had long periods with the same foster carers which, once ended, had led to a rapid turnover of unsatisfactory placements.

They were also more vociferous on the weaknesses of placements whether in foster or residential care. In one or two isolated cases foster care had worked well but in most cases foster placements had been an additional form of stress. One young woman referred graphically to the problems of entering someone's home to be confronted by a long list of rules and regulations. Some had been separated in early childhood from a sibling to whom they had been very close: one young woman was distressed by the fact that her foster family had refused to accept her brother because they only wanted to care for girls but had then gone on to adopt a boy. Others mentioned foster carers wanting them for company or for domestic duties and to a propensity for not treating them on an equal basis with their own children. More than half referred to abuse which they had suffered in a placement, usually with foster carers: only one mentioned violence and inhuman treatment which she had experienced in a children's home. Running away from placements was not uncommon; the distress was compounded by being returned to them. Notwithstanding, there was markedly less reporting of depression and self-harm than in the other group. With the exception of one who had become pregnant at the age of 13 and another who had done so at the age of 14, the young women in this group did not become pregnant at an earlier age then those in the group who became looked after in adolescence.

Sample of social workers and carers

Following the interview with the young person, contact was made with the social worker or carer whom they identified as being most involved in their case. In total 21 such workers were named and 20 were subsequently interviewed; the remaining one had a lengthy period of sick leave and had not returned to work at the end of the data collection period.

Of these, eight were social workers, seven were after-care workers, four were residential carers doing outreach work with young people who had been in residential care and one was a probation officer. The majority were women. In terms of location, one worker was from the north-east, ten from the north-west, eight from the central region and one from the south. In addition interviews took place with staff in supported accommodation for young women and with staff running groups for young mothers.

Component 2

Three locations were selected for the generation of the school sample. Census data (Office of Population Censuses and Surveys, 1994) and data from a recent Children's Services Plan indicate that the characteristics of the three areas are as follows:

Area A: Ward within a city. 7 per cent of young people from minority ethnic groups. Below national average for car ownership. Percentage of lone parents equivalent to national average.

Area B: Ward within a city. 9 per cent of young people from minority ethnic groups. High level of rented local authority accommodation (higher than national and city average). Below national and city average for car ownership. Above average number of lone parents.

Area C: Ward within a city. 38 per cent of young people from minority ethnic groups. High levels of rented local authority accommodation. Above average levels of lone parents.

Appendix B: Additional tables

Table A.1 Percentage agreeing with the following statements

	Looked after (%)			School (%)		
	Total	Male	Female	Total	Male	Female
If young people know the facts about sex and contraception it makes them more careful	73	78	68	78	82	73
It's easy being a father these days	23	18*	28	28	30	26
Young people have sex with their boy/girlfriend too early	69	61	78	81	79*	82
If young people know the facts about sex and contraception they are more likely to experiment	73	75.5	71*	61	71	50
It's easy for young people to get contraceptives	83	81	86	74	75.5	73
Young people today have a good future to look forward to	45	50	40	48	56	39.5
Women who carry condoms sleep around	23	33	14	27	39	14
My friends make me feel as though sex is the most important thing in a relationship	29	38	20	39	58*	16
Young men take their responsibilities seriously	39	61	19	45	63	24
I would be too embarrassed to talk to a new partner about contraception	39	43	35	36	42	29

Table A.2 Nikki and Kris vignettes

	Looked after (%)			School (%)		
	Total	Male	Female	Total	Male	Female
Nikki and Kris are both 15 and we have been going out together for two weeks. One of them wants to make this a sexual relationship. What do you think they should do?						
Go ahead now, if the other one agrees	35	44	26	32	41	19
Wait for another two weeks and think about it then	15	12	19	15	17	13
Wait six months	14	15	13	9	10	6
Wait until they are both 16	36	35	38	28	31	23
Go ahead now provided that they use contraception	38	48	28	36	41	30
Something else	13	4	23	25	14	38
They have agreed that this should become a sexual relationship. But in the meantime Nikki has discovered that Kris has been in trouble with the police over drugs and still does some drug dealing and house robberies. What should she do?						
End the relationship	38	33	42	33	31	34
Continue the relationship but tell him that the criminal behaviour must stop	38	39	37	52	56	47
Stay with him and try to change him	41	46	37	38	40	34
Continue to go out with him while she thinks about what to do	8	8	8	12	16	6
Carry on with the relationship because she's in love with him	16	21	12	14	19	9
Continue the relationship because she won't find anyone better	7	8	6	5	7	2
Continue because he's tough and will protect her	6	8	4	7	12	0
Something else	9	6	12	7	4	11
After having sex only once Nikki thinks she might be pregnant. How do you think she might feel?						
Worried about the future for herself and the baby	77	75	79	78	73	83
Happy	12	16	8	9	16	0
Anxious about telling her parents or carers	49	41	56	56	50	64
Worried about what her boyfriend would think	33	35	31	45	45	43
Wondering whether to have an abortion	36	39	33	60	55	66
Pleased because she knows she is able to have children	12	10	14	12	21	0
Something else	7	6	8	7	5	9

Table A.2 Continued

What do you think Nikki should do?	Looked after (%)			School (%)		
	Total	Male	Female	Total	Male	Female
Tell Kris	52	62	42	57	60	54
Get a pregnancy testing kit from the chemist's	62	64	60	68	72	63
Not worry because she wouldn't be pregnant the first time she had sex	9	6	12	7	9	4
Go and see her doctor	46	44	48	55	58	50
Tell her parents or carers	37	37	39	38	39	37
Go to the family planning clinic, advice clinic or Brook	44	40	48	47	44	50
Wait for another month before doing anything	15	12	19	12	7	17
Tell her best friend	32	27	37	38	35	41
Something else	7	6	8	3	4	2
She decides to tell Kris. How do you think he would feel?						
Great – he's going to be a father	23	33	13	11	19	0
Worried about what the future will look like	65	67	62	70	67	73
Annoyed that Nikki has got pregnant	23	17	28	37	33	41
Keen to tell his mates about it because they'll all be envious	25	35	15	26	26	4
Worried that Nikki might have an abortion	25	26	25	19	21	17
Anxious about telling his parents or carers	36	29	42	34	35	33
Hopeful that Nikki will have an abortion	21	16	26	51	53	48
Something else	11	8	13	8	11	4
Nikki and Kris have decided to keep the baby. Nikki's mother doesn't approve and tells her to leave. Nikki spends some time in care and some time with friends and always seems to be on the move. While this is going on she has to decide whether or not to stay on at school which she never really liked. What should she do?						
Leave straightaway because it's all too much and she probably wouldn't have got any GCSEs anyway	18	19	18	21	34	5
Try to find out if she can go to the school for pregnant schoolgirls	62	63	62	64	51	81
Carry on with her education and try to get some good exam results because she will need to get a good job later	54	48	60	69	72	65
Leave because Kris will get a job and look after her and the baby	17	21	14	19	26	11

Table A.2 Continued

	Looked after (%)			School (%)		
	Total	Male	Female	Total	Male	Female
Leave and go to college after she's had the baby	33	35	30	31	36	24
Something else	12	8	16	14	21	5
After a while she goes to live with Kris's family: his mother, stepfather and his two younger brothers in their 3-bedroomed house. Nikki and Kris share a small bedroom which they will also have to share with the baby. What should they do?						
Carry on living there but put their name on the housing waiting list	67	54	79	66	65	68
Move out to live with one of Kris's friends who lives with his girlfriend in a two-bedroomed flat which would give them more space but is damp and cold	11	8	15	16	20	11
Move out and become homeless so that the Council has to give them some sort of housing	21	23	21	22	37	3
Try to persuade Nikki's mother to take her and the baby while Kris lives with his mother	41	42	40	37	37	38
Something else	19	19	19	19	26	11
They've decided to carry on living in the cramped conditions at Kris's house and have had the baby who is now 3 months old. Kris wants to find a job and Nikki wants to go back to school. Who should look after the baby for the next year?						
Kris, while Nikki goes to school	29	27	31	32	41	20
Nikki, while Kris goes to work	24	28	20	17	24	9
Kris's mother, so that they can both do what they want to do	34	28	41	28	35	20
Nikki's mother	38	40	35	28	35	20
Kris's granny	19	17	20	25	30	17
Kris should go to work so they can pay for a childminder	27	34	20	28	36	31
Social Services should provide them with a free childminder	43	32	53	37	39	34
Something else	10	7	12	25	30	17

Index

abortion 5, 103–4, 115–21, 124, 187–88
abuse 136, 176
'accidents' 112–13
accommodation 163–73, 181–82, 191
   see also under specific types eg foster care
adoption 115–19, 124
after-care, see also leaving care
after-care centres 73
after-care workers 154–55, 157–59, 162, 189–90
age
   at first sexual intercourse 46–49
   at pregnancy 5, 148
alcohol 112
antenatal care 141–42, 189
aspirations 85–102, 186–87, 192–93
assessments 166

babies with disabilities 116
baby-sitting 169–70, 180
birth weight 10
boyfriends 47, 50–54, 131–33
   see also partners
Brook Advisory Centres 79, 120

carers 55, 184–86
   previous 159–61
   young people's views 32, 34–38, 40–41
   see also parents, social workers
child care 169–70, 180
childhood experiences 8, 15–17, 21–43, 85, 125–26,
   130, 143, 183–85
child-minding 169–70, 180
child protection 155, 157
Children Act (1989) 1–4, 60, 84, 149–50
Children Act, Guidance and Regulations 7, 58–59,
   82, 157
children in care see 'looked-after' children
children's homes, mother and baby in 166–67
Children's Society 150
choice 12
Choosing to Foster 60
cohabitation 6, 134
colleges 179–80
'comparator group' 15–20
condoms 72–74, 83
confidentiality 55
consultation 87–89
contraception 6–7, 61–62, 70–82, 106, 123, 186,
   193
   attitudes 70–71
   discussion with partner 81, 83–84
contraceptive services, access to 78–81
control 87–89
counselling 119–23
court orders 2

Department of Health 1
depression 10
deprived areas 6
drugs 112

early parenthood, young people's views 104–6,
   136–41
education 4, 89–94, 173–82, 191
   disruption 9, 58, 61, 91–92, 174
   during pregnancy 175–78
   young mothers 178–81
   see also schools
Education Act (1993) 57, 173
Education of Pupils Educated Otherwise than at
   School 173
emergency contraception 77–78
emotional influences 107–11
employment 23, 94–98, 134, 186
ethics 13
ethnic origins 18
Excellence in Schools 9
exclusion (from school) 175
expectations see aspirations

family background 21–27, 44
   see also childhood experiences
family centres 146–47, 190–91
family life 21–24, 42–43
   see also childhood experiences
fathers 6, 26–27, 115, 118, 131–36, 148
   see also parents, partners
financial help 134, 170–71
foster care 35, 38, 159, 165–66, 191
foster carers 3, 34–36, 59–60
friends 44–46, 56
further education see education

girlfriends 50–54
   see also partners

health 3–4, 10, 149, 189
Health of the Nation 1, 5
home tuition 177–78
housing 109–10, 157, 159, 167, 171–73
   see also accommodation

implants (contraceptive) 76–78
imprisonment 134–36
Independent Inquiry into Health Inequalities 2
independent living units 55, 150, 160, 171–73
injections (contraceptive) 76–78
'in public care' 2–4
interviews 13–20

joint parenting 129–36

leaving care 54, 149–51
    pregnant or as mothers 1, 8–9, 54, 183
    preparation 3–4, 11
living arrangements 6, 18
local authorities
    duties 1
    policies 11–12, 54–56, 58–61, 149–51, 163–66,
        188, 191–92
'looked after' children 2–4
'looked after' sample 15–20
Looking after Children 58–59, 78

magazines 68–69
marriage 98–102
morning-after pill 77–78
mother and baby units 55–56, 143–44, 151–57, 164,
        167, 169, 190–91
mothers 25–26, 29–31
    education 177–81
    see also parents

National Child Development Study 7
National Children's Homes 150
National Curriculum 9
National Foster Care association 165
National Task Group 2
New Ambitions for our Country 2

offenders 134–36
oral contraception 74–76
Our Healthier Nation 2, 183
outcomes 4

parent education 1, 9, 11, 23–24, 129, 148, 189
parenthood 125–49, 188–90
    coping with 141–47
    early 188–90
    expectations 125–29
    preparation for 125–49
    young people's views 100–101, 147–7
parenting 184
    joint 129–36
parenting ability 143–44
parents 24–32
    young people's views 27–33, 40–41
partners 6, 98–102
    see also fathers
peer pressure 48, 50–54, 56, 175, 185, 193
peer relationships 44–56
peers 185–86
pill see oral contraception
placement agreement meetings 60
policies, local authorities 11–12, 54–56, 58–61,
        149–51, 163–66, 188, 192
practical help 169–70
pregnancy
    attitudes to 81–82
    education during 175–78
    prevention 106
    reactions 113–15, 187–88
    reasons 6–9, 105–13, 123–24, 187
    termination see abortion
    views of others 110–11
    young people's views 103–24
'pregnancy schools' 175–77
preparation for adulthood 9
preparedness 11–12
pressure 106–7
previous carers 159–61
prosecutions 54

PSHE Advisory Group 9

Quality Protects 1, 4

racial origins 18
rape 108
reactions to pregnancy 113–15, 187–88
rejection 118–19, 124
relationships 90, 98–102, 131–33, 183–87, 190
    with adults 21–43
    with peers 44–56
religious beliefs 19, 46–47
residential care 32, 35–38
residential homes 35, 54, 160
    sexual relationships in 52–54
respect, from adults 40–42
rules 35, 168–69

sample 86–102
sample details 17–20, 199–211
school, absence 9, 58, 61, 91–92, 174
schools, sex education 57–58, 61–63
'school' sample 15–20
sex education 3, 6–7, 57–70, 82–84, 185–86
    in care 63–64
    effectiveness 66–70, 82–84
    from parents 64–66
    in schools 57–58
    young people's views 61–63, 66–70
sexual abuse 3, 8
sexual activity 55
sexual relationships 46–54, 185
    peer pressure 48, 185
    young people's views 48–50
siblings 21, 44, 184–85
significant adults 21–43
smoking 10
Social Exclusion Unit 2
social workers 12, 15, 20, 60–61, 151–57, 162, 184,
        190–91
    young people's views 38–41
    see also carers
socioeconomic status 7–8, 46
special units for education 175–77
study
    aims 11–12
    background 1–2, 12–20
support 9–15, 119–23, 141–47, 163–82, 190–92
supported accommodation 166–69
support groups 191
Supporting Families 2

teenage conceptions 54, 103–4
teenage fertility 5
teenage maternities 103–4
television 22–23, 68–69
training, in sex education 55, 59–60, 62–78
trust, from adults 40–42

under-age sex 46–50, 54–55

views, of young people 13
violence 22

When Leaving Home is Leaving Care 125
World Health Organisation 7

young mothers' groups 161
young parents, support for 149–62
youth clubs 15–17